Irena Roterman-Konieczna (Ed.)
Simulations in Medicine

Irena Roterman-Konieczna (Ed.)

Simulations in Medicine

Computer-aided diagnostics and therapy

DE GRUYTER

Editor
Prof. Dr. Irena Roterman-Konieczna
Department of Bioinformatics and Telemedicine
Jagiellonian University Medical College
Ul. Sw. Lazarza 16
31-530 Krakow
Poland
myroterm@cyf-kr.edu.pl

ISBN 978-3-11-066687-8
e-ISBN (PDF) 978-3-11-066721-9
e-ISBN (EPUB) 978-3-11-067691-4

Library of Congress Control Number: 2020931476

Bibliographic information published by the Deutsche Nationalbibliothek
The Deutsche Nationalbibliothek lists this publication in the Deutsche Nationalbibliografie; detailed
bibliographic data are available on the Internet at http://dnb.dnb.de.

© 2020 Walter de Gruyter GmbH, Berlin/Boston
Cover image: Eraxion / iStock / Getty Images Plus
Typesetting: Compuscript Ltd., Shannon, Ireland
Printing and binding: CPI books GmbH, Leck

www.degruyter.com

Foreword

Traditional medicine has, since its inception, registered numerous examples of treatment resulting in positive or negative outcomes, depending on the patient. This observation was reinforced after the completion of the human genome sequencing project. As it turns out, individual humans exhibit genetic differences despite possessing the same genome. The identification of so-called single nucleotide polymorphisms confirms and explains the familiar phenomenon of variable reaction to treatment [1, 2]. Given that even siblings differ in terms of their chromosomal material, the genetic variability of the general human population should come as no surprise. Recent research has also revealed differences in the composition of gut bacterial flora resulting from diverse dietary habits [3]. In light of such specificities, the need for individual, personalized therapy becomes evident. Fortunately, many high-tech tools can be used in medical practice (Chapter 1).

The most direct applications of personalized medicine involve individualized pharmacotherapy. Drugs designed to interact with a specific target may help improve therapeutic outcomes while remaining affordable, particularly in the presence of bioinformatic technologies. Identifying links between molecular chemistry and pathological processes is among the goals of system biology [4]. Access to computer software that simulates the complete proteome may help discover causal reactions—not just in the scope of a particular disease, but between seemingly unconnected processes occurring in the organism [4]. Harnessing the power of modern computers in an objective, dispassionate therapeutic process will enhance the capabilities of medical practitioners, for example, by offering access to vast databases of biological and medical knowledge (Chapter 2). Moreover, processing data with the use of artificial intelligence algorithms may lead to conclusions which a human would not otherwise be able to reach (Chapter 2).

Closer collaboration between communication system experts and biologists should help identify promising research directions and explain the methods by which organisms—the most complex biological systems known to man—identify and process information (Chapter 3).

Gaining insight into the molecular phenomena will help resolve some long-standing fundamental questions. Even before this happens, however, medical science can reap benefits by exploiting existing solutions and models (Chapter 4).

Eliminating transplant rejection is of critical importance in individualized therapy. Three-dimensional bioprinting technologies represent an important milestone on this path (Chapter 5). They can be used to build arbitrarily complex objects, with local variations in the applied materials. An advanced printing environment may enable introduction of biological material (e.g., cells harvested from the patient for whom the implant is being created) directly at the printing stage (Chapter 5). Similarly, the shape of the printed tissue may accurately reflect the patient's needs, which

https://doi.org/10.1515/9783110667219-202

is particularly important, e.g., when recreating the layout of coronary vessels for bypass surgery.

Surgeons may also benefit greatly from the use of robots that surpass humans in their capacity to perform repetitive actions with great accuracy (Chapter 6).

Modern diagnostic tools that both simplify the therapeutic process and improve its accuracy already provide added value for doctors. A hybrid operating room that supports both macro- and microscale (cellular) activities enhances on-the-fly decision making during surgery (Chapter 7).

Recent advances in augmented reality technologies are finding their way into the operating theater, assisting surgeons and enabling them to make the right choices as the surgery progresses. Holographically superimposing imaging results (such as CAT scans) on the actual view of the patient's body (made possible by AR headsets) enhances the surgeon's precision and eliminates errors caused by inaccurate identification of the surgical target (Chapters 8 and 9).

The use of computers in medical research also encompasses the organization system of a hospital. The software monitoring information and transport of materials (as well as medical equipment) in hospital units delivers the logistic system for the communication of patients and doctors in medical practice (Chapter 10).

The medical treatment takes advantage of applying the techniques of telecommunication, allowing the conduct of therapy and especially surgery independently between medical doctors participating in the therapeutic practice from a distance (Chapter 11).

Medical education implements the training simulation using phantoms. The computer-based steering of phantom behavior allows the medical students to be familiar with the patient's behavior in extreme conditions, conscienceless, or rising emotions (Chapter 12).

This publication should be regarded as an extension of our previous work, presenting the use of simulation techniques in studying systems of variable structural complexity (including the human organism [5]). The overview presented simulations carried out at several scales, from individual molecules, through cells and organs, all the way to the organism as a whole.

The simulation of diagnostic processes is presented with the use of so-called virtual patients, whereas therapeutic approaches are discussed on the example of chemotherapy. We also present psychological aspects related to gamification and describe 3D printing as a means of treating skeletal defects. In this hierarchy of ever-greater involvement of IT technologies, the final tier is occupied by telemedicine. All tiers are discussed against the backdrop of preclinical activities described in the previous edition of *Simulations in Medicine*.

The current overview focuses on the use of simulation techniques in clinical practice and decision support, particularly in delivering personalized therapeutic solutions. Personalized therapy is currently the focus of significant research effort in areas such as genomics, epigenetics, drug design, and nutrition, while also yielding practical benefits, such as those described in the presented work. The subject has engendered numerous publications, some of which are explicitly mentioned in our study.

Both editions of *Simulations in Medicine* demonstrate the extensive practical applications of *in silico* solutions. The marriage of medicine and information science promises to result in tools and approaches that facilitate large-scale adoption of personalized therapy. It seems, however, that the effective design of personalized treatment options calls for better understanding of processes such as protein folding and 3D structure prediction. Pathologies that affect the folding process lead to a variety of medical conditions jointly referred to as misfolding diseases. This phenomenon is among the most pressing challenges facing modern medical research [6–18].

References

[1] Vogenberg FR, Isaacson Barash C, Pursel M. Personalized medicine. "Part 1: evolution and development into theranostics." *Pharmacy and Therapeutics* 35, no. 10 (2010): 560–76.

[2] Brittain HK, Scott R, Thomas E. "The rise of the genome and personalised medicine." *Clinical Medicine (London)* 17, no. 6 (2017): 545–51. doi:10.7861/clinmedicine.

[3] Gentile CL, Weir TL. "The gut microbiota at the intersection of diet and human health." *Science* 362 (2018): 776–80.

[4] Konieczny L, Roterman-Konieczna I, Spólnik P. *Systems Biology.* Springer, 2012.

[5] Roterman-Konieczna I. *Simulations in Medicine.* de Gruyter, 2015.

[6] Jackson SE, Chester JD. "Personalised cancer medicine." *International Journal of Cancer* 137, no. 2 (2015): 262–6. doi:10.1002/ijc.28940.

[7] Almeida A, Kolarich D. "The promise of protein glycosylation for personalised medicine." *Biochimica et Biophysica Acta* 1860, no. 8 (2016): 1583–95. doi:10.1016/j.bbagen.2016.03.012.

[8] O'Brien JM. "Personalised medicine-the potential yet realised." *BJOG* 125, no. 3 (2018): 351. doi:10.1111/1471-0528.14846.

[9] Lee ST, Scott AM. "Nuclear medicine in the era of personalised medicine." *Journal of Internal Medicine* 48, no. 5 (2018): 497–9. doi:10.1111/imj.13789.

[10] Doble B, Schofield DJ, Roscioli T, Mattick JS. "The promise of personalised medicine." *Lancet* 387, no. 10017 (2016): 433–4. doi:10.1016/S0140-6736(16)00176-8.

[11] Carrasco-Ramiro F, Peiró-Pastor R, Aguado B. "Human genomics projects and precision medicine." *Gene Therapy* 24, no. 9 (2017):551–61. doi:10.1038/gt.2017.77.

[12] Maggi E, Montagna C. "AACR precision medicine series: highlights of the integrating clinical genomics and cancer therapy meeting." *Mutatation Research* 782 (2015): 44–51. doi:10.1016/j.mrfmmm.2015.10.005.

[13] Tian Q, Price ND, Hood L. "Systems cancer medicine: towards realization of predictive, preventive, personalized and participatory (P4) medicine." *Journal of Internal Medicine* 271, no. 2 (2012): 111–21. doi:10.1111/j.1365-2796.2011.02498.x.

[14] Brall C, Schröder-Bäck P. "Personalised medicine and scarce resources: a discussion of ethical chances and challenges from the perspective of the capability approach." *Public Health Genomics* 19, no. 3 (2016): 178–86. doi:10.1159/000446536.

[15] Maughan T. The promise and the hype of 'personalised medicine'. *New Bioethics* 23, no. 1 (2017): 13–20. doi:10.1080/20502877.2017.1314886.

[16] Krittanawong C, Zhang H, Wang Z, Aydar M, Kitai T. Artificial intelligence in precision cardiovascular medicine. *Journal of the American College of Cardiology* 69, no. 21 (2017): 2657–64. doi:10.1016/j.jacc.2017.03.571.

[17] Matuchansky C. "The promise of personalised medicine." *Lancet* 386, no. 9995 (2015): 742. doi:10.1016/S0140-6736(15)61541-0.

[18] Al-Metwali B, Mulla H. "Personalised dosing of medicines for children." *Journal of Pharmacy and Pharmacology* 69, no. 5 (2017): 514–24. doi:10.1111/jphp.12709.

Kraków September 2019

Irena Roterman-Konieczna
Department of Bioinformatics and Telemedicine
Jagiellonian University Medical College

Contents

Foreword —— v
Contributing authors —— xv

Patryk Orzechowski, Michael Stauffer, Jason H. Moore,
and Mary Regina Boland
1   Personalized medicine —— 1
1.1   Introduction —— 1
1.2   Three-dimensional printing —— 3
1.2.1   Medical 3D bioprinting —— 4
1.2.2   Medical devices —— 4
1.2.3   Anatomical models for surgery planning —— 5
1.2.4   Medication manufacturing —— 5
1.3   Holography and personalized medicine —— 6
1.3.1   Holographic sensors and point-of-care testing —— 6
1.3.2   Holographic sensors and surgery —— 7
1.4   Robotics —— 7
1.5   Computer modeling —— 8
1.6   Hybrid operating room —— 8
1.6.1   Hybrid OR —— 9
1.6.2   Augmented, virtual, and extended reality (AR/VR/XR) —— 9
1.6.3   VR for visualization and assessment of mitral valve geometry
           in structural heart disease —— 10
1.6.4   3D-ARILE by the Fraunhofer Institute for Computer Graphics Research
           IGD —— 11
1.7   Summary —— 11
1.8   References —— 12

Krzysztof Kotowski, Piotr Fabian, and Katarzyna Stapor
2   Machine learning approach to automatic recognition of emotions based on
           bioelectrical brain activity —— 15
2.1   Introduction —— 15
2.2   Psychological models of emotion —— 16
2.3   EEG correlates of emotion —— 19
2.3.1   Event-related potentials —— 19
2.3.2   Spectral density (frequency domain) —— 20
2.4   Introduction to machine learning —— 21
2.4.1   The concept of machine learning —— 21
2.4.2   The importance of data sets —— 22
2.5   Automatic emotion recognition using machine learning —— 22
2.5.1   Sources of the data —— 22

2.5.1.1   EEG data sets —— **23**
2.5.1.2   EEG simulators —— **23**
2.5.1.3   Custom EEG experiments —— **25**
2.5.2   Methods —— **26**
2.5.2.1   Preprocessing —— **26**
2.5.2.2   Feature extraction —— **27**
2.5.2.3   Emotion classification and estimation using
           machine learning —— **27**
2.5.3   Results —— **28**
2.5.4   Applications —— **28**
2.6   Summary —— **30**
2.7   Acknowledgments —— **30**
2.8   References —— **30**

Grzegorz Marcin Wójcik
3   **Selected methods of quantitative analysis**
           in electroencephalography —— **35**
3.1   Introduction —— **35**
3.2   EEG technology and resting state —— **36**
3.3   EEG rhythms and power spectrum —— **38**
3.4   Event-related potentials —— **39**
3.5   Dipole source modeling —— **39**
3.6   Source localization LORETA/sLORETA —— **40**
3.7   Principal component analysis —— **42**
3.8   Independent component analysis —— **42**
3.9   Software reviews —— **43**
3.9.1   OpenSesame —— **43**
3.9.2   Net Station —— **44**
3.9.3   GeoSource —— **46**
3.9.4   EEG lab —— **47**
3.9.5   Brainstorm —— **47**
3.10   Example of the Iowa Gambling Task experiment —— **48**
3.11   Where do we go from here? —— **53**
3.12   References —— **53**

Anna Sochocka, Liwia Leś, and Rafał Starypan
4   **The visualization of the construction of the human eye** —— **55**
4.1   Introduction —— **55**
4.2   Overview of the existing solutions —— **56**
4.3   Presentation of the written application —— **57**
4.4   Summary —— **62**
4.5   References —— **62**

Jan Witowski, Mateusz Sitkowski, Mateusz K. Hołda,
and Michał Pędziwiatr

5   **Three-dimensional printing in preoperative
         and intraoperative decision making** —— **63**
5.1   Introduction —— **63**
5.2   Introduction of 3D printing to clinical practice —— **63**
5.3   The 3D printing process —— **64**
5.4   Clinical example: liver models —— **66**
5.5   Clinical example: congenital heart disease and transcatheter
             interventions —— **67**
5.6   Creating in-house 3D lab and summary —— **69**
5.7   References —— **71**

Zbigniew Nawrat

6   **Virtual operating theater for planning Robin Heart robot operation** —— **73**
6.1   Introduction —— **73**
6.2   Introduction to surgical operation —— **73**
6.3   Modeling and planning of a surgical procedure —— **74**
6.4   Training —— **78**
6.5   Planning of robotic operations —— **81**
6.6   Robin Heart —— **82**
6.7   Exercises with students —— **86**
6.8   Summary —— **90**
6.8.1   Robots and virtual space technologies —— **90**
6.9   References —— **93**

Piotr Mazur, Maciej Bochenek, Krzysztof Bartuś, Roman Przybylski,
and Bogusław Kapelak

7   **Hybrid room: Role in modern adult cardiac surgery** —— **95**
7.1   Introduction —— **95**
7.2   Components of the hybrid room —— **95**
7.2.1   Surgical requirements —— **95**
7.2.2   Room requirements —— **96**
7.2.3   Fixed C-arm and imaging techniques —— **96**
7.2.4   Image fusion —— **97**
7.2.5   Radiation safety —— **97**
7.2.6   Training —— **97**
7.3   Clinical application of the hybrid room —— **98**
7.3.1   TAVI —— **98**
7.3.2   Hybrid coronary artery revascularization —— **99**
7.3.3   Endovascular aortic repair —— **100**
7.3.4   Hybrid antiarrhythmic procedures —— **100**

7.4   Conclusions —— **100**
7.5   References —— **101**

Klaudia Proniewska, Damian Dołęga-Dołęgowski,
Agnieszka Pręgowska, Piotr Walecki, and Dariusz Dudek
8   **Holography as a progressive revolution in medicine —— 103**
8.1   Introduction to holographic technology —— **103**
8.2   Augmented reality versus virtual reality —— **104**
8.3   AR, VR, and holograms for the medical industry —— **107**
8.4   Training and mode of action scenarios—medical VR/AR —— **107**
8.5   Teaching empathy through AR —— **108**
8.6   Holography in the operating room —— **110**
8.7   Medical holographic applications—our team examples —— **112**
8.7.1   A wireless heart rate monitor integrated with HoloLens —— **112**
8.7.2   Holography in stomatology —— **114**
8.8   Future perspectives: visualization of anatomical structures —— **115**
8.9   References —— **115**

Joanna Szaleniec and Ryszard Tadeusiewicz
9   **Robotic surgery in otolaryngology —— 117**
9.1   Introduction —— **117**
9.2   General remarks —— **119**
9.3   Robotic surgery in head and neck—advantages
          and disadvantages —— **119**
9.4   Applications of the da Vinci system for head and neck surgery —— **123**
9.5   Transoral robotic operations —— **124**
9.6   The FLEX system —— **125**
9.7   Conclusion —— **125**
9.8   References —— **125**

Jan Witowski, Mateusz Sitkowski, Mateusz K. Hołda,
Michał Pędziwiatr and Marek Piotrowski
10   **Hospital management —— 128**
10.1   Hybrid rooms —— **128**
10.2   Integrated rooms —— **129**
10.3   Surgical robotics —— **131**
10.4   Patient verification systems —— **137**
10.5   Management systems for surgical instruments —— **138**
10.6   Intensive medical care area management system —— **140**
10.7   Medical device management systems —— **143**
10.8   Radio- and brachytherapy management systems —— **148**

Tomasz Rogula, Aneta Myszka, Tanawat Vongsurbchart,
and Nasit Vurgun

11   Robotic surgery training, simulation,
       and data collection ── 150
11.1   History and progress of training in minimally
           invasive surgery ── 150
11.2   Simulation and training with respect to robotic surgery ── 154
11.2.1   Training ── 154
11.2.2   Simulation ── 155
11.2.3   VR simulators ── 155
11.2.4   Physical training ── 157
11.3   Robotic courses ── 157
11.3.1   Fundamentals of robotic surgery ── 157
11.3.2   Robotics Training Network (RTN) ── 159
11.3.3   SAGES Robotics Masters Series ── 159
11.3.4   Fundamental skills of robot-assisted surgery (FSRS)
           training program ── 160
11.3.5   da Vinci Technology Training Pathway ── 160
11.4   Early clinical training in robotic surgery ── 161
11.5   Global data collection for robotic surgery ── 162
11.6   References ── 165

Grzegorz Cebula and Michał Nowakowski
12   Simulation in medical education—phantoms in medicine ── 168
12.1   Introduction ── 168
12.2   Full-body simulators application in the training
           of medical personnel ── 169
12.2.1   History ── 169
12.3   The capabilities of different types of simulators ── 169
12.3.1   Partial body simulators ── 170
12.3.2   Nursing care simulators ── 171
12.3.3   Advances life support full-body simulator essential properties ── 172
12.3.4   Advanced patient simulators ── 173
12.3.5   Virtual reality and enhanced reality simulators ── 174
12.3.5.1   Virtual reality ── 174
12.3.5.2   Enhanced/augmented reality ── 174
12.4   Nontechnical skills training ── 175
12.4.1   Crisis resource management ── 175
12.4.1.1   Situation awareness ── 176
12.4.1.2   Cognitive errors ── 176
12.4.1.3   Planning and decision making ── 177
12.4.2   Teamwork ── 178

12.4.2.1   The 10-seconds-for-10-minutes technique—sharing decision making —— **178**
12.4.2.2   Team leader skills —— **178**
12.4.2.3   Communication —— **179**
12.4.2.4   Close loop communication —— **179**
12.4.2.5   Team member's name use during communication —— **179**
12.4.2.6   Team assertiveness —— **179**
12.4.3   Technical skills training —— **180**
12.4.3.1   See one, do one, teach one —— **181**
12.4.3.2   Peyton four-step approach —— **181**
12.4.3.3   Slicing method/skill deconstruction —— **182**
12.4.3.4   Programmatic teaching of technical skills —— **183**
12.5   Summary —— **183**
12.6   References —— **183**

Index —— **185**

Contributing authors

Krzysztof Bartuś
Institute of Cardiology
Jagiellonian University Medical College
Pradnicka St. 80
31-202 Kraków
Poland
krzysztofbartus@gmail.com

Department of Cardiovascular Surgery and
Transplantology
John Paul II Hospital
Kraków
Poland

Maciej Bochenek
Department of Heart Transplantation and
Mechanical Circulatory Support
Wroclaw Medical University
Borowska St. 213
50-556 Kraków
Poland
bochenekmd@gmail.com

Mary Regina Boland
Institute for Biomedical Informatics
University of Pennsylvania
Philadelphia, PA 19104
USA

Department of Biostatistics, Epidemiology
and Informatics
University of Pennsylvania
Philadelphia, PA 19104
USA

Center for Excellence in Environmental
Toxicology
University of Pennsylvania
Philadelphia, PA 19104
USA

Department of Biomedical and Health
Informatics
Children's Hospital of Philadelphia
Philadelphia, PA 19104
USA

Grzegorz Cebula
Department of Medical Education
Jagiellonian University Medical College
Kraków
Poland

Damian Dołęga-Dołęgowski
Department of Bioinformatics and Telemedicine
Jagiellonian University Medical College
Kopernika 7e
31-034 Kraków
Poland
dolegadolegowski@gmail.com

Dariusz Dudek
Department of Interventional Cardiology
University Hospital
Jagiellonian University Medical College
Kopernika 17
31-501 Kraków
Poland
mcdudek@cyfronet.pl

Piotr Fabian
Institute of Informatics
Silesian University of Technology
Akademicka 2a
44-100 Gliwice
Poland
piotr.fabian@polsl.pl

Mateusz K. Hołda
Department of Anatomy
Jagiellonian University Medical College
Kopernika 12
31-034 Kraków
Poland
mkh@onet.eu

Bogusław Kapelak
Institute of Cardiology
Jagiellonian University Medical College
Pradnicka St. 80
31-202 Kraków
Poland
bogus.kapelak@gmail.com

Department of Cardiovascular Surgery and
Transplantology
John Paul II Hospital
Kraków
Poland

Krzysztof Kotowski
Institute of Informatics
Silesian University of Technology
Akademicka 2a
44-100 Gliwice
Poland
krzysztof.kotowski@polsl.pl

Liwia Leś
Faculty of Physics, Astronomy and Applied
Computer Science
Łojasiewicza 11
30-059 Kraków
Poland

Piotr Mazur
Institute of Cardiology
Jagiellonian University Medical College
Kraków
Poland
piotr.k.mazur@gmail.com

John Paul II Hospital
Department of Cardiovascular Surgery and
Transplantology
Pradnicka St. 80
31-202 Kraków
Poland

Jason H. Moore
Institute for Biomedical Informatics
University of Pennsylvania
Philadelphia, PA 19104
USA

Department of Biostatistics, Epidemiology and
Informatics
University of Pennsylvania
Philadelphia, PA 19104
USA

Aneta Myszka
Department of Surgery
Jagiellonian University Medical College
ul. Jakubowskiego 2
30-688 Kraków
Poland
anetamyszka95@gmail.com

Zbigniew Nawrat
Department of Biophysics,
School of Medicine with the Division
of Dentistry in Zabrze
Medical University of Silesia
Jordana 19
41-808 Zabrze
Poland
www.biofiz.sum.edu.pl

Professor Zbigniew Religa Foundation
of Cardiac Surgery Development
Institute of Heart Prostheses
Wolności Str. 345a, 41-800 Zabrze
Poland

Michał Nowakowski
2nd Chair of Surgery
Jagiellonian University Medical College
Kraków
Poland

Patryk Orzechowski
Institute for Biomedical Informatics
University of Pennsylvania
Philadelphia, PA 19104
USA
patryk.orzechowski@gmail.com

Department of Biostatistics, Epidemiology
and Informatics
University of Pennsylvania
Philadelphia, PA 19104
USA

Department of Automatics and Robotics
AGH University of Science and Technology
al. A. Mickiewicza 30
30-059 Kraków
Poland

Michał Pędziwiatr
2nd Department of General Surgery
Jagiellonian University Medical College
Kopernika 21
31-501 Kraków
Poland
michal.pedziwiatr@uj.edu.pl

Marek Piotrowski
University Hospital, Department of
Medical Equipment
Kopernika 19
31-501 Kraków
Poland

Agnieszka Pręgowska
Institute of Fundamental Technological Research
Polish Academy of Sciences
Pawinskiego 5B
02-106 Warsaw
Poland
aprego@ippt.pan.pl

Klaudia Proniewska
Department of Bioinformatics and Telemedicine
Jagiellonian University Medical College
Kopernika 7e
31-034 Kraków
Poland
klaudia.proniewska@uj.edu.pl

Roman Przybylski
Department of Heart Transplantation and
Mechanical Circulatory Support
Wroclaw Medical University
Borowska St. 213
50-556 Kraków
Poland
romanprzybylski@o2.pl

Tomasz Rogula
Department of Surgery
Jagiellonian University Medical College
ul. Jakubowskiego 2
30-688 Kraków
Poland
tomasz.rogula@uj.edu.pl

BrainX EU–Research Group for Surgical AI
Jagiellonian University Medical College
Kraków
Poland

Mateusz Sitkowski
2nd Department of General Surgery
Jagiellonian University Medical College
Kopernika 21
31-501 Kraków
Poland
mateusz.sitkowski@alumni.uj.edu.pl

Anna Sochocka
Faculty of Physics, Astronomy and Applied
Computer Science
Department of Game Technology
Jagiellonian University
Łojasiewicza 11
30-059 Kraków
Poland
anna.sochocka@uj.edu.pl

Katarzyna Stąpor
Institute of Informatics
Silesian University of Technology
Akademicka 2a
44-100 Gliwice
Poland
katarzyna.stapor@polsl.pl

Rafał Starypan
Private scientist
rapast@poczta.fm

Michael Stauffer
Institute for Biomedical Informatics
University of Pennsylvania
Philadelphia, PA 19104
USA

Department of Biostatistics, Epidemiology and
Informatics
University of Pennsylvania
Philadelphia, PA 19104
USA

Joanna Szaleniec
Department of Otolaryngology
Jagiellonian Univesity Medical College
Jakubowskiego 2
30-688 Kraków
Poland
joanna.szaleniec@uj.edu.pl

Ryszard Tadeusiewicz
Chair of Biocybernetics and Biomedical
Engineering
AGH University of Science and Technology
Al. Mickiewicza 30
30-059 Kraków
Poland
rtad@agh.edu.pl

Tanawat Vongsurbchart
Department of Surgery
Jagiellonian University Medical College
ul. Jakubowskiego 2
30-688 Kraków
Poland
tanawatv19@gmail.com

Nasit Vurgun
Department of Surgery
Jagiellonian University Medical College
ul. Jakubowskiego 2
30-688 Kraków
Poland
nasitv@gmail.com

Piotr Walecki
Department of Bioinformatics and Telemedicine
Jagiellonian University Medical College
Kopernika 7e
Pradnicka St. 80
31-034 Kraków
Poland
piotr.walecki@gmail.com

Jan Witowski
2nd Department of General Surgery
Jagiellonian University Medical College
Kopernika 21
31-501 Kraków
Poland
jan.witowski@alumni.uj.edu.pl

Grzegorz Marcin Wójcik
Maria Curie-Sklodowska University in Lublin
Faculty of Mathematics, Physics and Computer
Science
Institute of Computer Science
Chair of Neuroinformatics and Biomedical
Engineering
ul. Akademicka 9
20-033 Lublin
Poland

Patryk Orzechowski, Michael Stauffer, Jason H. Moore, and
Mary Regina Boland

1 Personalized medicine

1.1 Introduction

Everyone is different. Each person represents a unique combination of genomic, demographic, developmental, occupational, and environmental factors. This also means that treatment challenges for every person are not the same.

Traditional medicine is based on the application of protocols. If a given therapy was observed to be successful for a group of people in a randomized controlled trial (RCT), then traditional medicine concludes that the treatment should work for all patients. Although this assumption works in general, with recent scientific advancements, it has become clear that there are situations where the assumptions fail because of the following reasons.

First, traditional approaches do not account for the ethnic heterogeneity of patients. The risks for developing many diseases vary across ethnic groups. In addition to disparities in disease risk across races and ethnicities, there are also survival disparities across different racial groups (e.g., 5-year survival rates among those with breast cancer) [1–4].

Second, the one-protocol-to-heal-them-all approach does not necessarily account for confounding factors, such as race, age, gender, body mass index, socioeconomic status, or even birth month [5–8]. Protocols impose an "if-else" rule-based approach, which usually depends on the observation of laboratory tests and the response of the patient to the treatment. In addition, most clinical protocols are based on initial RCTs. However, in order for an RCT to be adequate, all possible confounders need to be identified *a priori* before the randomization occurs. If one confounder variable is missing during the randomization step, then the results of the RCT would not generalize to those groups.

Third, there is a diversity of patients' responses to treatment. A higher response rate to the treatment for a group of people may also be associated with increased toxicity for the other. This basically means that even if a given treatment helps some people or subpopulation of the study, the treatment may be harmful to another subpopulation.

There is also the issue of adherence to the treatment regime. Certain patient populations do not believe in taking prescription medications because of ideological reasons (e.g., those adhering to the scientology religion do not believe in taking prescription medications). Therefore, RCTs may exclude these individuals because they are not willing to cooperate with the treatment protocol. However, in some cases, these individuals still enter hospitals and seek medical care. If this patient subpopulation has never participated in any clinical RCTs, it may be difficult to determine whether the treatment would be effective among this patient population. They are essentially an unstudied patient population. These constitute some of the very important and critical challenges faced by personalized and precision medicine in the twenty-first century.

An important concern is that many clinical trials are not representative of the diversity that exists in human populations. For example, Kwiatkowski et al. [9] studied ethnic and gender diversity in 304 publications between 2001 and 2010 and found out that in 277 treatments and 27 prevention trials, over 80% of participants were white and nearly 60% were male. Another study by Chen et al. [10] pointed out that the percentage of reporting minorities from five major studies in literature varied between 1.5% and 58.0%, and only 20% of papers in high impact factor oncology journals detailed the results broken down by each separate ethnic group. There is an ongoing effort to encourage minorities to participate in random clinical trials [11]. However, this is a challenging area because researchers must overcome years of mistrust generated by a system that has often been discriminatory toward minority populations [12]. To conclude, efforts need to be made to redesign clinical trials to reflect the diversity of the patient population treated in the clinic and to address issues pertaining to individuals themselves instead of populations as a whole.

The aforementioned challenges with traditional approaches in medicine show an emerging need for developing more customizable treatments based on the "true" patient [13], which would be more fit to a given patient, instead of focusing on general outcome statistics [14]. Schork [15] reported that somewhere between 1 in 25 and 1 in 4 (25%) patients are actually receiving benefit from taking some of the most popular drugs in the United States. For example, statins, which are prescribed to lower cholesterol, were said to benefit only 1 in 50 patients.

As in personalized medicine, there are no historical data for each of the patients; therefore, recent efforts focus on tailoring treatment to a given set of characteristics of the patient rather than to the entire individual as a whole. Precision medicine is about giving the right patient the right drug in the right dosage at the right time [16]. Tailoring a therapy based on the observation of the context of the patient allows therapy adjustments down to a fine-grained level of detail. The hope is that this would improve the prognosis and reduce costs of the treatment.

In recent years, there has been a noticeable increase in interest on the implementation of precision medicine programs. The "All of Us" initiative was launched in the United States in 2015 with the aim to recruit at least one million individuals with diverse lifestyles, environments, and biology to create a database for scientific analysis that is open to researchers around the world. Similar programs, but on a smaller scale, were also launched across the globe: Australia, Belgium, Canada, Estonia, France, Israel, Japan, Korea, Luxembourg, Singapore, Thailand, and the United Kingdom [17]. Much of the effort is taken to create as accurate data as possible, including multiomic data, i.e., genomic, proteomic, transcriptomic, epigenomic, microbiomic, and other information. The combined data could be analyzed to search for patterns for common diseases. By combining knowledge about the patient, not only disease prognosis could be predicted, but also its susceptibility of the disease and the patient's response to certain treatments. This research could lead to an improvement in the health and outcome of the patient.

Similarly, an individualized approach can support better understanding of genetic factors for rare diseases. A rare disease is defined by the Food and Drug Administration (FDA) as a disease, affecting fewer than 200,000 people in the United States (≥0.06%). The FDA has identified a total of 7,000 diseases meeting these rare disease criteria, many of which have no known treatment.[1] Understanding molecular mechanisms in different diseases could create a better classification of diseases. This can allow researchers to repurpose existing drugs used for treating one disease for treatment in another [18].

The volume of health care-specific data is increasing. The number and amount of publicly available data sets is rapidly growing. The Database of Genotypes and Phenotypes offers access to both publicly available and restricted individual level data [19, 20]. The Gene Expression Omnibus created in 2000 stores more than 40,000 data sets with 1,200,000 of samples by 2018 [21–23]. Creating repositories with collected biological samples (biobanking) as well as the integration of multiple types of data (multiomics) has provided different sources of information. This multiview approach could allow better understanding of mechanisms of diseases.

With a growing number of publicly available patient data, there is an emerging need to implement novel techniques for data analysis. With recent advances in machine learning, deep learning becomes widely used in biomedical sciences [24]. Another technique that has become more popularly applied to bioinformatics is biclustering [25]. This data mining technique can be used to identify subgroups of patients with specific characteristics [26, 27]. With the recent progress in the field and development of sophisticated and accurate methods that can extract informative patterns, a step was made toward finding explanation for diseases [28–31].

In the subsequent parts of this chapter, we provide a very brief introduction into different techniques and their applications to personalized medicine.

1.2 Three-dimensional printing

Printing in 3D, which is a process of building a 3D object layer by layer based on a computer model [32], has already allowed rapid prototyping and customization in manufacturing, designing, and production of parts for automation or components

---

1 www.fda.gov/industry/developing-products-rare-diseases-conditions/rare-disease-day-2019.

for construction. This technique was invented in the early 1980s by Charles Hull and called "stereolithography." The exact processes of 3D printing differ and depend on the material used, device, speed, or resolution [33].

One of the first reported applications of 3D printing in medical domain was the development of prosthetics and dental implants [34]. Since then, 3D printing has made a great impact on medicine by allowing the development of customized bones, ears, cells, blood vessels, tissues, or even organs. This area of application is called bioprinting. Three-dimensional printing has also allowed the emergence of multiple personalized medical devices as well as drug development.

In this part, we overview the recent applications of 3D printing technology in medicine.

1.2.1 Medical 3D bioprinting

Enabling 3D printing of biocompatible materials could be considered a recent breakthrough in regenerative medicine. The integration of multiple technologies from biomaterial sciences, engineering, cell biology, medicine, and physics has allowed to deliver synthetic cells or tissues, including a multilayered skin, bone, or even heart [35, 36]. This provides a technique for the creation and development of cells or even organs in biosynthetic materials, which could be later transplanted to patients. With high need for tissues and organs for transplantation, biocompatible materials could be used as a potential alternative. The implantation of cells or organs that would mimic the native ones in both geometry and cell distribution has been sought for over a decade. The rejection rate might be minimized by using cells from the donor's own body, which could serve to create a replacement organ [33, 37].

A typical process of 3D bioprinting begins with imaging of the damaged tissue, choosing the design (biomimicry, self-assembly, or minitissue building blocks), selecting the material (the most popularly used materials are synthetic or natural polymers or decellularized Extracellular matrix (ECM)) and cells, bioprinting, and application, which either could be in vitro or may require some maturation in a bioreactor before it could be transplanted [36].

1.2.2 Medical devices

The personalization of the medical devices has played a great role especially in cases where the patient is expected to be wearing a device for an extended period. One of the success stories of the application of 3D printing in health care is manufacturing hearing aids. The process of fitting the right hearing aids used to be handcrafted and was very lengthy. In the situation where a millimeter of difference in the design of a device could cause discomfort to the patient, 3D printing comes with the perfect aid. By imaging, a device could be perfectly fitted to the patient, which greatly shortens the process and improves the comfort [33].

Another example of using a personalized device for improving health care is the Invisalign® aligner [38]. The set of orthodontic devices allowing a gentle adjustment of teeth location has proven to successfully help thousands of patients without the necessity to wear visible braces.

The development of personalized masks for acne treatment is another interesting application of 3D printing. By taking a digital image of a patient's face, a mask is manufactured, which allows to dissipate the solution evenly on the skin of the patient [39].

1.2.3 Anatomical models for surgery planning

What is even more promising is that computer models can be printed using 3D printers, which could increase the success rate of very complex surgeries. In this way, the surgical removal of tumor from involved organs could be practiced in a simulator as needed before the actual procedure, without any harm to the patient. Similarly, vascular modeling may enable cardiac surgeons to implant stents customized to the patient. A digital model of the blood vessels can serve to design the stents of the proper construction: size, shape, and bendability. The stent could be later printed and implanted to the patient with greater success rate than the conventional ones and decrease rejection rate [31].

1.2.4 Medication manufacturing

One of the latest trends in using 3D printing for biomedicine is the development of targeted drugs or those with different release times. The first 3D-printed drug called Spritam® was approved by the FDA in 2015. The drug offers treatment for seizures in epilepsy [39].

A 3D-printed drug has been successfully used as a patch for the prolonged release of anticancer drug in pancreatic cancer treatment [40]. This allows the drug to reach desirable concentration at the tumor sites, in contrast to traditional chemotherapeutic drugs, which are poorly soluble in aqueous media.

There is ongoing research on creating multidrug pills. Those personalized pills would substitute multiple pills administered to a patient with a single personalized pill. Patients would no longer need to remember the dosages of different drugs, e.g., two pills of one drug three times per day and one pill of another drug twice a day.

Instead, a simplified pill would be administered, and all the required doses would be released automatically. This should improve the car by minimizing the mistakes of the patients, such as taking too much pills of a first drug or missing another [33].

1.3 Holography and personalized medicine

Holograms have been popularized in science fiction and often consist of a 3D image that interacts with a user when triggered (e.g., when an individual walks up to a kiosk). But what are holograms, and how can they be used to advance personalized medicine? Holograms are 3D images that are formed by the interference of light beams from a laser or other coherent light source [41]. Holography is the science and study of making holograms.

So how can holograms be used in personalized or precision medicine? By definition, holograms are made through the interference of light beams that produces an image. Holographic sensors are sensors that change color based on the angle of light that refracts from the structure. They consist of 3D analyte nanostructures. When the light diffracts from these nanostructures, one can learn something informative about what is taking place [41].

1.3.1 Holographic sensors and point-of-care testing

For example, there are colorimetric urine tests that measure pH, protein, and glucose in patients' urine. A smartphone algorithm was also developed to quickly read the results of these colorimetric tests and to detect important color changes in the urine in response to the test [42]. This would be especially useful for those that are color blind and unable to read the color change results themselves.

Colorimetric tests are an emerging area of point-of-care medicine [43]. These tests have been suggested as proof of concepts for blood-based biomarker tests for psychiatric diseases [44]. They could be used to detect if a patient is having a chemical imbalance crisis event, which is important in psychiatric disease treatment. These point-of-case colorimetric tests could also be used to detect if patients are taking their prescription medications (drug adherence) or using illicit substances [45]. Biometric holography can also be used to detect chemoresistance among patients [46].

Environmental exposures, such as exposure to DDT (an insecticide used to reduce the mosquito population), could also be monitored via colorimetric tests, which have been described as early as the 1940s [47] but are gaining more traction recently [48]. These colorimetric methods would be very useful in the future to help quantify the number and kinds of environmental exposures. A recent study on prenatal exposures found that at least 219 distinct environmental exposures have been studied in the literature with regard to their prenatal effects [6]. Therefore, methods are needed to easily identify if individuals have been exposed to these various exposures, and if so, to what extent.

1.3.2 Holographic sensors and surgery

Microsoft has developed a new HoloLens in which researchers are developing methods in the surgical context. Holographic methods can be used to detect and clearly delineated cancerous from noncancerous tissue. However, it is often difficult to implement these methods in the surgical context because of surgeons' reliance on their natural eyesight to make important delineations that may not be captured by current digital methods. Therefore, rather than fully replacing a surgeon's eyesight with a digital headset, researchers are beginning to use Microsoft's HoloLens to augment the surgeons natural eyesight without fully replacing their eyes to help in delineating cancerous from noncancerous tissue [49]. These methods are still in their nascent stages, and much work is required in this area to make these methods applicable and usable in the clinical setting.

1.4 Robotics

One of the areas used to be thought of as science fiction and has now become a reality is robot-assisted surgery. Over 1.75 million robotic procedures have been performed in the last 14 years in the United States only [50].

Robotics can improve health care by supporting aid at minimal invasive surgeries. Robotic arm could be much more precise than a human hand and better control surgery instruments. It also does not transmit tremors manned surgeries. This allows for more precise operations, smaller incisions, and decreased loss of blood. As the results of postsurgery complications risks are usually decreased, hospitalization shortened and recovery process speeded up.

One of the robotic devices that have already become established is the *da Vinci* robot by Intuitive Surgical. The robot, operated from the console, was approved by the U.S. FDA for performing different complex medical surgeries that support gynecology, urology, and other disciplines. It is commonly used worldwide for prostatectomies and gynecologic surgeries. Similar devices are also developed by other companies.

Intensive work is also being done on remote surgeries, which could be performed by a skilled specialist from any place in the world. According to *PC Magazine*, the first successful remote operation on a human using 5G network was performed in China.[2] The surgeon who was located over 1,800 miles from the operating room implanted

---

2 https://www.dailymail.co.uk/health/article-6821613/Surgeon-performs-world-remote-brain-surgery-patient-1-800-MILES-AWAY.html.

deep brain stimulation device to a patient suffering from Parkinson's disease. With the rapid development of 5G mobile network, such surgeries may become more popular and improve local health care, especially in cases when transportation of the patients is unsafe or expensive.

Although the progress in robotics is clearly visible, multiple challenges still remain. A nonnegligible number of surgical complications were observed. Among over 1.75 million of robotic-assisted surgeries performed between 2000 and 2013, among 10,624 reported adverse events, 144 deaths, 1,391 patient injuries, and 8,061 device malfunctions were reported [50].

1.5 Computer modeling

One of the ways how recent technologies change reality is computer modeling. In the recent years, simulation has moved far beyond classic approaches for visualizing large data sets [51]. Digital models of certain organs or tissues acquired using visualization techniques, such as CT, MRI, X-ray, or ultrasound, could be used as simulators, which can be used to train future generation of surgeons. Similarly, performing a procedure on a real patient is no longer the only way that surgeons may learn their profession. The 3D-printed physical models of real organs may serve as a great educational tool for surgeons.

Visualization technologies bring also a deeper insight into the actual nature of a particular disorder. Creating a digital model of an actual organ of a patient may allow to better understand the nature of a particular disorder. Different reparative procedures could be compared, and thus the optimal procedure or treatment could be adjusted to the patient. Digital copies of the organ may also be shared and discussed by a group of physicians.

Another area of interest is modeling a patient within the health system. With digitalization, electronic health records were introduced in multiple providers across Europe and the United States. The major aim of the systems was storing patients' data in digital forms, which included all procedures, physicians' notes, and laboratory results. With the expansion of data mining and machine learning, electronic systems became invaluable sources of information. Unfortunately, the systems were not designed for this purpose, and the extraction of data is sometimes challenging. Different approaches are made to better understand the interaction of patients with the health care. For example, by modeling trajectories of patients for different diseases, groups with different survival chances may be extracted, which could be later used for targeting similar patients with different treatments [52].

1.6 Hybrid operating room

The way that surgeries are performed has significantly changed over the last few years. With access to more advanced technologies, diagnostics, and imaging, increasingly complex procedures are performed and—what is even more spectacular—are successful in delivering the proper care to the patient.

In this section, we start with a short overview of a modern surgical theater, which is called a hybrid operating room (OR). We also highlight some of the recent advances in techniques of extended reality and the ways that it has started to be adapted in operating theaters. A more thorough information on hybrid OR could be found in Chapter 7 of this book.

1.6.1 Hybrid OR

The quality of surgeries is continuously increasing, thanks to the better training of the surgeons, as well as the investments in facilities by hospital stakeholders. Combining a traditional OR with interventional suite with advanced imaging and visualization creates a space for more advanced surgeries. This facility, usually operated by an interdisciplinary team of clinicians, is also called a hybrid OR.

Hybrid ORs are modern spaces that facilitate state-of-the-art equipment, allowing image-guided or minimal invasive procedures or even open procedures. Instant access to C-arms, CT, or MRI devices during the procedure allows constant monitoring of the state and instantaneous adjustment during the procedure. This is especially valuable for providing the best care for patients undergoing cardiac or neurovascular procedures.

The flexibility offered by hybrid ORs is not limited to cardiac or neurosurgeries. With access to such advanced facilities, the facilities can also provide support for ER, laparoscopic, orthopedic trauma surgeries, and many others.

1.6.2 Augmented, virtual, and extended reality (AR/VR/XR)

Virtual reality (VR) and augmented reality (AR) technologies, collectively called extended reality (XR), have been in development and use since the 1990s but have recently become much more affordable and much easier to work with, and developing software for these applications has become easier as well. Because of this, there is a boom in new XR applications, and there is a fast growth in adoption across many fields, including health care, data visualization, gaming, architecture, and training and maintenance within many fields. Within health care, some applications fit within the broader topic of personalized medicine.

The difference between VR and AR lies in the relationship between the computer-generated virtual experiences and the real world. In VR, a user is completely immersed in a virtual world. Typically, this is achieved by wearing a head-mounted display capable of stereographic image projection that completely blocks out the user's view of the real world. Two well-known systems of this type are the HTC Vive and the Oculus Rift. Interaction with the virtual world typically involves two handheld controllers that the user manipulates. The application can completely control the world that the user sees and interacts. In AR systems, the user wears a headset with a see-through projection screen, sometimes in the form of what looks like glasses. The computer-generated imagery is projected into the user's eyes from this screen and overlaid on top of the user's view of the real world. In contrast to VR, AR allows the user to navigate and interact with the real world while viewing computer-generated imagery.

The following are some examples of surgical XR applications. Other examples of how personalized medicine could be used for a hybrid OR may be found in Chapter 7 of the book.

1.6.3 VR for visualization and assessment of mitral valve geometry in structural heart disease

In this small study, the SyGlass[3] VR application is evaluated as a tool to assist in the modeling and measurement of mitral valve (MV) geometry [53]. The long-term goal of the project is to develop an easier and faster method for evaluating the MV geometry of a patient with MV anomalies. There are two common MV anomalies, each addressed by a different surgical procedure. The geometry of the MV determines which procedure should be used, and the echocardiogram that is used to image the valve is performed at the beginning of the patient's time in the OR. Thus, there is a need for a quick and easily learned method to analyze the patient's MV geometry in the OR.

Conventionally, interactive 3D modeling of the MV in echocardiography involves visualizing and interacting with the valve in a volume-rendered image and a series of cross-sectional planes on a standard 2D computer display. Although this is a state-of-the-art method, it requires a sophisticated 2D-to-3D mental integration step to identify and measure individual components of the MV, it is time consuming, and it requires specialized training. By contrast, the SyGlass application presents a 3D volume of the MV in VR, which allows for much more natural perception of and interaction with the 3D structure. The user can look around naturally to get different views of the MV, yielding very rich depth and structural information. They can hold a virtual marker tool in their hand and reach out naturally to line it up precisely in space with the portion of the MV they intend to mark for specifying its geometry.

This preliminary study suggests that the use of SyGlass for MV measurement has reproducible high accuracy, and it is quick. If further study confirms these findings, this method could be performed on site in the OR to help make a quick decision about which surgical procedure to implement for the patient.

---

3 syglass.io.

1.6.4 3D-ARILE by the Fraunhofer Institute for Computer Graphics Research IGD

The 3D-ARILE system[4] is an experimental AR system meant to assist in the surgical removal of a sentinel lymph node after the excision of a malignant melanoma tumor. A near infrared-activated dye is injected in the lymph node, and a custom 3D NIR-sensitive camera tracks its location in space. The surgeon wears a custom AR headset that interacts with the 3D camera to collect information about the lymph node's position in space and then presents an image of the lymph node to the surgeon, overlaid on the patient's body. The surgeon can change her move, and the overlaid lymph node image maintains its proper representation in space. Because AR allows the surgeon to view the virtual lymph node image overlaid on the real-world image of the patient, she has a more natural 3D view of the lymph node and can work directly on the surgical site without having to change her view to an external monitor. This promises greater accuracy and speed during the tumor excision.

1.7 Summary

For the last couple of years, personalized medicine has made enormous progress to deliver better, faster, and more customizable treatment to multiple patients. By taking an individualized, nonstandard approach, better fitting solutions could be proposed to the patients, and thus the time and cost of providing improper treatment could be saved.

Multiple advances were adapted in health care throughout the last decade. The progress was observed in imaging (e.g., more precise 3D images of organs, and emergence of sophisticated extended reality devices), prosthetics, orthodontics or orthopedics (3D-printed implants), drug design and transplantation (3D bioprinting), and modeling vessels or organs. The advances in robotics have started to allow fully remote surgeries, which will become even more popular with the implementation of 5G network across the countries. Hybrid ORs, which are becoming more popular in the modern hospitals, have already allowed clinicians to perform very advanced medical procedures. The progress in robotics justify thinking of unmanned (i.e., fully autonomous) surgeries in the future.

Personalized medicine cannot be narrowed down to a specific method or application. It should be considered as a multidisciplinary approach, which puts the health of the patient in the first place and offers advanced options for the recovery in modern facilities. This shift in approach from "follow the protocol" to individualized therapy requires a holistic approach, which will simultaneously consider the nature

---

4 www.fraunhofer.de/en/press/research-news/2017/november/ar-glasses-help-surgeons-when-operating-on-tumors.html.

of the patients' problems and previous expert knowledge on treatments that could be helpful for the particular person.

In this book, a closer look into multiple areas of personalized medicine is taken. With this short introductory, we overviewed some of the most interesting applications of personalized medicine. The more detailed information on the selected techniques could be found in the subsequent parts of this book.

1.8 References

[1] Amorrortu, Rossybelle P, et al. "Recruitment of racial and ethnic minorities to clinical trials conducted within specialty clinics: an intervention mapping approach." *Trials* 19 (2018): 115.

[2] Burroughs, Valentine J, Randall W. Maxey, Richard A. Levy. "Racial and ethnic differences in response to medicines: towards individualized pharmaceutical treatment." *Journal of the National Medical Association* 94.10 Suppl (2002): 1.

[3] Settle, Kathleen, et al. "Racial survival disparity in head and neck cancer results from low prevalence of human papillomavirus infection in black oropharyngeal cancer patients." *Cancer Prevention Research* 2.9 (2009): 776–81.

[4] Wikoff, William R, et al. "Pharmacometabolomics reveals racial differences in response to atenolol treatment." *PloS One* 8.3 (2013): e57639.

[5] Boland MR, Shahn Z, Madigan D, Hripcsak G, Tatonetti NP. "Birth month affects lifetime disease risk: a phenome-wide method." *Journal of the American Medical Informatics Association* 22 (2015): 1042–53.

[6] Boland MR, et al. "Uncovering exposures responsible for birth season–disease effects: a global study." *Journal of the American Medical Informatics Association* 25 (2017): 275–88.

[7] Boland MR, Kraus MS, Dziuk E, Gelzer AR. "Cardiovascular disease risk varies by birth month in Canines." *Scientific Reports* 8 (2018): 7130.

[8] Boland MR, Kashyap A, Xiong J, Holmes J, Lorch S. "Development and validation of the PEPPER framework (Prenatal Exposure PubMed ParsER) with applications to food additives." *Journal of the American Medical Informatics Association* 25 (2018): 1432–43.

[9] Kwiatkowski, Kat, et al. "Inclusion of minorities and women in cancer clinical trials, a decade later: have we improved?" *Cancer* 119 (2013): 2956–63.

[10] Chen Jr, Moon S, et al. "Twenty years post-NIH Revitalization Act: enhancing minority participation in clinical trials (EMPaCT): laying the groundwork for improving minority clinical trial accrual: renewing the case for enhancing minority participation in cancer clinical trials." *Cancer* 120 (2014): 1091–6.

[11] Hamel, Lauren M, et al. "Barriers to clinical trial enrollment in racial and ethnic minority patients with cancer." *Cancer Control* 23 (2016): 327–37.

[12] Durant RW, Legedza AT, Marcantonio ER, Freeman MB, Landon BE. "Different types of distrust in clinical research among whites and African Americans." *Journal of the National Medical Association* 103 (2011): 123–30.

[13] Boland MR, Hripcsak G, Shen Y, Chung WK, Weng C. "Defining a comprehensive verotype using electronic health records for personalized medicine." *Journal of the American Medical Informatics Association* 20 (2013): e232–8.

[14] Lu, Yi-Fan, et al. "Personalized medicine and human genetic diversity." *Cold Spring Harbor Perspectives in Medicine* 4 (2014): a008581.

[15] Schork, Nicholas J. "Personalized medicine: time for one-person trials." *Nature News* 520 (2015): 609.

[16] Roberts, Jason A, Anand Kumar, Jeffrey Lipman. "Right dose, right now: customized drug dosing in the critically ill." *Critical Care Medicine* 45 (2017): 331–6.

[17] Ginsburg, Geoffrey S, Kathryn A. Phillips. "Precision medicine: from science to value." *Health Affairs* 37 (2018): 694–701.

[18] Schee Genannt Halfmann S, Mählmann L, Leyens L, Reumann M, Brand A. "Personalized medicine: what's in it for rare diseases?" In: Posada de la Paz M, Taruscio D, and Groft S, eds. *Rare Diseases Epidemiology: Update and Overview. Advances in Experimental Medicine and Biology*, Vol. 1031. Switzerland: Springer, 2017.

[19] Mailman, Matthew D, et al. "The NCBI dbGaP database of genotypes and phenotypes." *Nature genetics* 39 (2007): 1181.

[20] Tryka, Kimberly A, et al. "NCBI's database of genotypes and phenotypes: dbGaP." *Nucleic Acids Research* 42 (2013): D975–9.

[21] Clough, Emily, Tanya Barrett. "The gene expression omnibus database." *Statistical Genomics*, pp. 93–110. New York: Humana Press, 2016.

[22] Edgar, Ron, Michael Domrachev, Alex E. Lash. "Gene expression omnibus: NCBI gene expression and hybridization array data repository." *Nucleic Acids Research* 30 (2002): 207–10.

[23] Wang, Zichen, Alexander Lachmann, Avi Ma'ayan. "Mining data and metadata from the gene expression omnibus." *Biophysical Reviews* 11 (2019): 103–10.

[24] Ching, Travers, et al. "Opportunities and obstacles for deep learning in biology and medicine." *Journal of the Royal Society Interface* 15 (2018): 20170387.

[25] Xie, Juan, et al. "It is time to apply biclustering: a comprehensive review of biclustering applications in biological and biomedical data." *Briefings in Bioinformatics* 1 (2018): 16.

[26] Orzechowski, Patryk, Krzysztof Boryczko. "Propagation-based biclustering algorithm for extracting inclusion-maximal motifs." *Computing and Informatics* 35 (2016): 391–410.

[27] Orzechowski, Patryk, Krzysztof Boryczko, Jason H. Moore. "Scalable biclustering—the future of big data exploration?" *GigaScience* 8 (2019): giz078.

[28] Gusenleitner, Daniel, et al. "iBBiG: iterative binary bi-clustering of gene sets." *Bioinformatics* 28 (2012): 2484–92.

[29] Orzechowski, Patryk, et al. "Runibic: a bioconductor package for parallel row-based biclustering of gene expression data." *Bioinformatics* 34 (2018): 4302–4.

[30] Orzechowski, Patryk, et al. "EBIC: an evolutionary-based parallel biclustering algorithm for pattern discovery." *Bioinformatics* 34 (2018): 3719–26.

[31] Orzechowski, Patryk, Jason H. Moore. "EBIC: an open source software for high-dimensional and big data analyses." *Bioinformatics* (2019): btz027. https://doi.org/10.1093/bioinformatics/btz027.

[32] Sachs, Emanuel, et al. "Three dimensional printing: rapid tooling and prototypes directly from a CAD model." *Journal of Engineering for Industry* 114 (1992): 481–8.

[33] Ventola, Lee C. "Medical applications for 3D printing: current and projected uses." *Pharmacy and Therapeutics* 39 (2014): 704.

[34] McGurk M, et al. "Rapid prototyping techniques for anatomical modelling in medicine." *Annals of the Royal College of Surgeons of England* 79 (1997): 169.

[35] Kolesky, David B, et al. "3D bioprinting of vascularized, heterogeneous cell-laden tissue constructs." *Advanced Materials* 26 (2014): 3124–30.

[36] Murphy, Sean V, Anthony Atala. "3D bioprinting of tissues and organs." *Nature Biotechnology* 32 (2014): 773.

[37] Cohen, Daniel L, et al. "Direct freeform fabrication of seeded hydrogels in arbitrary geometries." *Tissue Engineering* 12 (2006): 1325–35.

[38] Wong, Benson H. "Invisalign A to Z." *American Journal of Orthodontics and Dentofacial Orthopedics* 121 (2002): 540–1.

[39] Konta, Andrea, Marta García-Piña, Dolores Serrano. "Personalised 3D printed medicines: which techniques and polymers are more successful?" *Bioengineering* 4 (2017): 79.

[40] Yi, Hee-Gyeong, et al. "A 3D-printed local drug delivery patch for pancreatic cancer growth suppression." *Journal of Controlled Release* 238 (2016): 231–41.

[41] Yetisen AK, Naydenova I, da Cruz Vasconcellos F, Blyth J, Lowe CR. "Holographic sensors: three-dimensional analyte-sensitive nanostructures and their applications." *Chemical Reviews* 114 (2014): 10654–96.

[42] Yetisen AK, Martinez-Hurtado JL, Garcia-Melendrez A, da Cruz Vasconcellos F, Lowe CR. "A smartphone algorithm with inter-phone repeatability for the analysis of colorimetric tests." *Sensors and Actuators B: Chemical* 196 (2014): 156–60.

[43] Vashist SK, Luppa PB, Yeo LY, Ozcan A, Luong JH. "Emerging technologies for next-generation point-of-care testing." *Trends in Biotechnology* 33 (2015): 692–705.

[44] Guest FL, Guest PC, Martins-de-Souza D. "The emergence of point-of-care blood-based biomarker testing for psychiatric disorders: enabling personalized medicine." *Biomarkers in Medicine* 10 (2016): 431–43.

[45] Argente-García A, Jornet-Martínez N, Herráez-Hernández R, Campíns-Falcó P. "A solid colorimetric sensor for the analysis of amphetamine-like street samples." *Analytica Chimica Acta* 943 (2016): 123–30.

[46] Choi H, Li Z, Sun H, Merrill D, Turek J, Childress M, Nolte D. "Biodynamic digital holography of chemoresistance in a pre-clinical trial of canine B-cell lymphoma." *Biomedical Optics Express* 9 (2018): 2214–28.

[47] Stiff HA, Castillo JC. "A colorimetric method for the micro-determination of 2, 2, bis (p-chlorophenyl) 1, 1, 1 trichlorethane (DDT)." *Science* 101(1945): 440–3.

[48] Ismail HM, et al. "Development of a simple dipstick assay for operational monitoring of DDT." *PLoS Neglected Tropical Diseases* 10 (2016): e0004324.

[49] Cui N, Kharel P, Gruev V. "Augmented reality with Microsoft HoloLens holograms for near infrared fluorescence based image guided surgery." In: *Molecular-Guided Surgery: Molecules, Devices, and Applications III*. Vol. 10049, p. 100490I. International Society for Optics and Photonics, 2017.

[50] Alemzadeh, Homa, et al. "Adverse events in robotic surgery: a retrospective study of 14 years of FDA data." *PloS One* 11 (2016): e0151470.

[51] Orzechowski, Patryk, Krzysztof Boryczko. "Parallel approach for visual clustering of protein databases." *Computing and Informatics* 29 (2012): 1221–31.

[52] Beaulieu-Jones, Brett K, Patryk Orzechowski, Jason H. Moore. "Mapping patient trajectories using longitudinal extraction and deep learning in the MIMIC-III Critical Care Database." *Pacific Symposium on Biocomputing* 23 (2018): 123–132.

[53] Aly HA, et al. "Virtual reality for visualization and assessment of mitral valve geometry in structural heart disease." *Circulation* Suppl. (in press).

Krzysztof Kotowski, Piotr Fabian, and Katarzyna Stapor

2 Machine learning approach to automatic recognition of emotions based on bioelectrical brain activity

Abstract: The feeling and the expression of emotions are the basic skills of social interaction. People with disorders such as autism, attention deficit/hyperactivity disorder, or depression may experience social marginalization because of problems with these skills. Automatic emotion recognition systems may help in diagnosis, monitoring, and rehabilitation. Specific patterns of bioelectrical brain activity in response to affective stimuli (facial expressions, music, and videos) are biomarkers of perceived emotions. The analysis of these patterns in the time domain (event-related potentials) or frequency (brain waves) is complicated because of the scale and complexity and our incomplete knowledge about the processes taking place in the brain. Nowadays machine learning methods, including deep learning, come with help along with the growing amount of available data. In this study, the state-of-the-art methods for the recognition of emotions based on electroencephalography data will be presented.

2.1 Introduction

The most common way of measuring bioelectrical brain activity is electroencephalography (EEG). It is a completely noninvasive and relatively cheap method used in brain-computer interfaces, cognitive psychology, and medical diagnostics. The EEG electrodes placed on the scalp record the electrical activity between groups of neurons in the cortical surface of the brain. It enables the EEG practitioners to find patterns of this activity connected with certain actions, disorders, and mental states. PubMed reports over 168,000 publications related to EEG. The great number of them is connected with the diagnosis of epilepsy and the prediction of epileptic seizures as the most popular applications of EEG in medicine [1, 2]. The second very popular area is anesthesiology, where the EEG is used to assess the depth of anesthesia and to monitor the effects of psychotropic drugs and anesthetic agents [3, 4]. Finally, the last wide, emerging area of the main interest in this publication is connected with the diagnostics of mental disorders such as autism spectrum disorder (ASD) [5], attention deficit/hyperactivity disorder (ADHD) [6], schizophrenia [7, 8], depression [9], dementia [10], or sleep disorders [11].

Many mental disorders are characterized by problems connected with the right feeling and expression of emotions. People with ASD, ADHD, or depression, especially when not diagnosed early, may experience social marginalization because of these problems. Psychotropic drugs, like antidepressants, and antipsychotics, work by interfering with the monoamine system, which is essential in the control of behaviors and emotions according to many studies [12]. At the same time, the emotions themselves are an important factor in the regulation of a human's mental and physical health. As stated by Luneski *et al.* [13], positive emotions may provide health benefits by accelerating the recovery of patients after heart surgery, having cardiovascular diseases or breast cancer, and are able to increase the level of salivary immunoglobulin (S-IgA). By contrast, negative emotions may weaken the human immune system, increase the risk of common cold up to four times [14], and reactivate the latent Epstein-Barr virus [15]. Thus, a significant motivation exists for researching emotions and minimizing their effect on specific aspects of human health.

However, the patterns of EEG connected with mental disorders and emotions are noisy, inconclusive, and hard to capture even for experts in the field. Thus, the EEG in psychiatry is usually considered a method of a low detection rate and a low diagnostic yield [10]. This is where computer science and computational methods (like machine learning) may come to help increase the reliability of existing procedures and discover the new ones when dealing with complexities of the human brain. Computing that relates to, arises from, or influences emotions is defined as affective computing [16].

This chapter presents the state-of-the-art computer-aided emotion recognition methods and their applications in practice, with special focus on the medical context. It starts with an introduction to the theoretical models of emotions and their EEG correlates. Chapter 2.4 defines the term machine learning and explains how the computer is able to learn from the provided data. Chapter 2.5 presents the whole process of emotion recognition using machine learning, including literature review, data collection, feature extraction, classifiers, and results analysis. In addition, the short review of EEG simulators is included.

2.2 Psychological models of emotion

Analysis of emotions or emotional states needs to be preceded with the definition of the model in which they are measured. Our emotions are mental states generated by the central nervous system [17]. Despite a number of significant works, emotion theory is still far from complete. Human emotions are, to a large extent, subjective and nondeterministic. The same stimulus may create different emotions in different individuals, and the same individual may express different emotions in response to the same stimulus, at different times. Despite this variability, it is assumed that there are basic principles, perhaps even basic neural mechanisms, that make a particular event "emotional" [16]. There are a number of emotional state space models, generally categorized into discrete and continuous models.

The discrete emotion models describe different numbers of independent emotion categories. One of the most popular models by Paul Ekman [18] describes six universal basic emotions of anger, disgust, fear, happiness, sadness, and surprise. The model is derived from the observation of universal facial expressions presented in Fig. 2.1. The paper describing the model [18] has been cited over 7,000 times; however, the existence of basic emotions is still an unsettled issue in psychology, rejected by many researchers [19]. Another model by Plutchik [20] describes eight primary bipolar emotions: joy and sadness; anger and fear; surprise and anticipation; and trust and disgust. However, unlike Ekman's model, Plutchik's wheel of emotions relates these pairs in the circumplex model. Recently, the model consisting of as many as 27 classes bridged by continuous gradients was proposed [21].

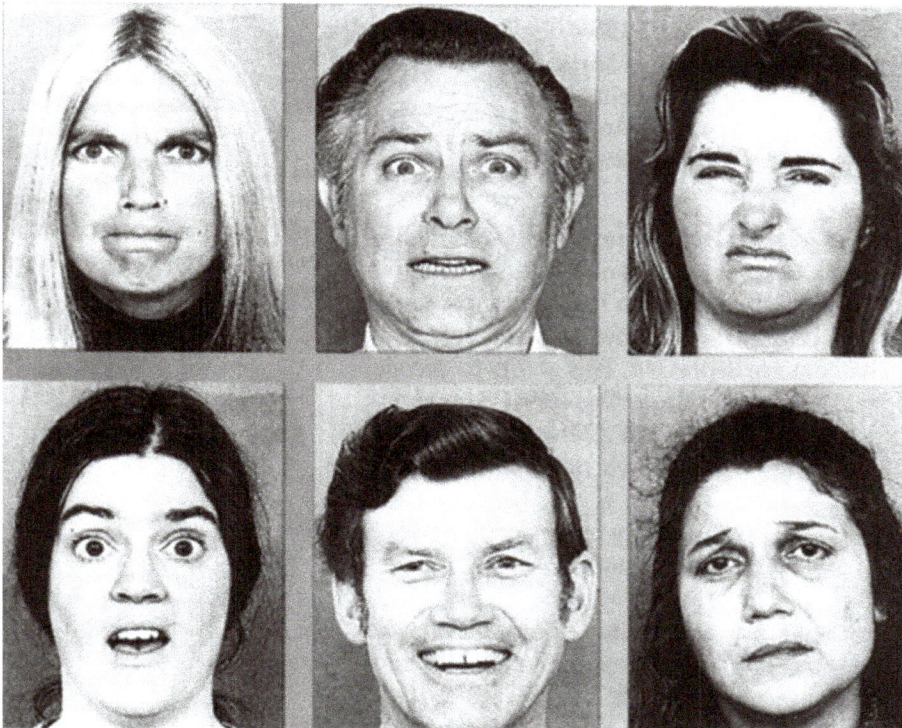

Fig. 2.1: Facial expressions of six basic Ekman emotions. Top row: anger, fear, and disgust. Bottom row: surprise, happiness, and sadness.

The continuous models are usually represented in numerical dimensional space. The most popular dimensions were defined by Mehrabian and Russell [22] as pleasure, arousal, and dominance (PAD model). The first dimension is frequently called *valence* in the literature; it describes how pleasant (or unpleasant) is the stimuli for the participant. The arousal dimension defines the intensity of emotion. Dominance is described as a level of control and influence over one's surroundings and others [23]. Usually, less attention is paid to this third dimension in the literature [24]. However, only the dominance dimension enables to distinguish between angry and anxious, alert and surprised, or relaxed from protected [23]. The model that includes only valence and arousal levels is called a circumplex model of affect [25] and is one of the most commonly used to describe the emotions elicited with stimuli. Various adjectives may be assigned to specific values of valence and arousal, as shown in Fig. 2.2 (i.e., a state of high arousal and high valence may be described as the state of excitement). For purposes of emotion classification, the model is sometimes discretized by defining four subspaces of LALV, LAHV, HALV, and HAHV on the ranges of valence and arousal (as shown in Fig. 2.1), where LAHV means low-arousal high-valence subspace. There are also works on full mappings between different discrete and continuous emotion models [26].

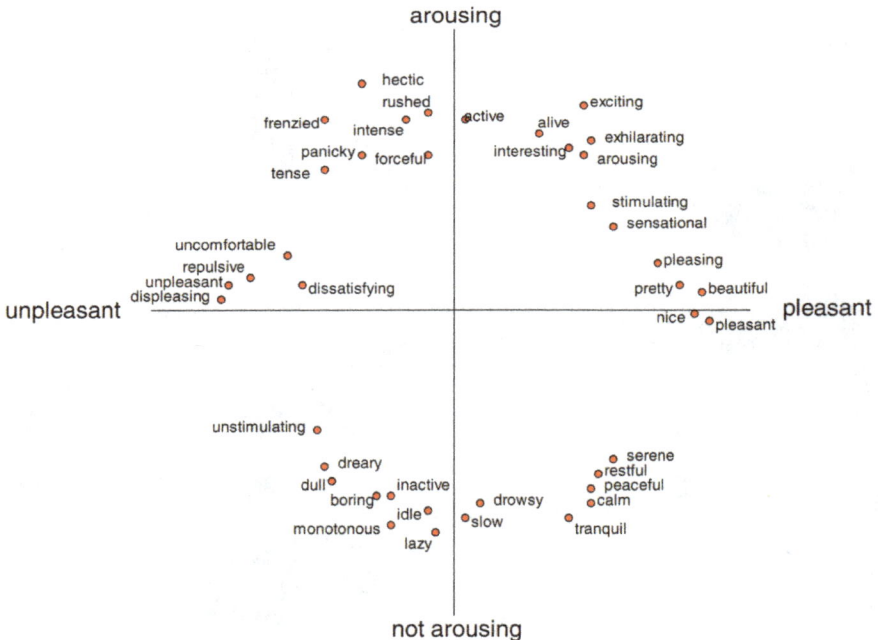

Fig. 2.2: The circumplex model of affect as presented by Russell *et al.* [25].

2.3 EEG correlates of emotion

The relation between EEG data and current emotional state may be considered in the context of two main approaches: the locationist and the constructionist paradigms. The locationist approach is closely related to the theory of basic emotions described in chapter 2.2. It assumes that each emotion is generated by a unique neural pathway and has a unique footprint in brain signal [18]. Similarly to the theory of the basic emotions, the locationist approach is currently being criticized by many researchers in the field [27]. They present the constructionist approach as the alternative where the emotions result from the interaction of different functional networks of the brain. There is some recent evidence that using dimensional models derived from the constructionist approach (like PAD) reflects the brain activity by means of EEG data more coherently [28]. Also, the majority of recent papers in automatic emotion recognition use dimensional models [29].

Different stimuli may be used to induce specific emotions and their correlates. Typically, the normative sets of videos, images, music, and/or odors are used. They are provided with emotional ratings obtained from a large population using self-assessment forms. The most common image set of this kind is the International Affective Picture System (IAPS) [30].

The number of studies has shown that correlates of emotion are usually associated with event-related potentials (ERPs), frontal EEG asymmetry, event-related synchronization, and steady-state visually evoked potentials (for reviews, see [29, 31]).

2.3.1 Event-related potentials

The ERPs are the stereotyped brain responses elicited by specific stimuli. They are analyzed in the time domain as waveforms composed from a number of components of different latency and amplitudes. The modulation of these latencies and amplitudes in the context of emotional processing has been analyzed for more than 50 years. Affective stimuli affect mainly the amplitudes of the components [32]. The earlier ERP components of latency up to 300 ms have been shown to correlate more with the valence dimension, i.e., by enhanced N100 (negative amplitude component with 100 ms latency) and N200 components' amplitude for unpleasant stimuli. These effects have been theoretically associated with attention orientation at early stages of processing. Also, it has been shown that unpleasant and high arousing stimuli evoke greater ERP responses for females relative to males [33]. The arousal dimension is reflected by later components N200, P300, and slow waves (550 to 850 ms after stimuli onset) with higher amplitudes for more arousing stimuli [34]. The basic emotions processing is frequently analyzed by means of ERP correlates of facial expression perception. Here, the early posterior negativity (EPN, in the range of 240–340 ms)

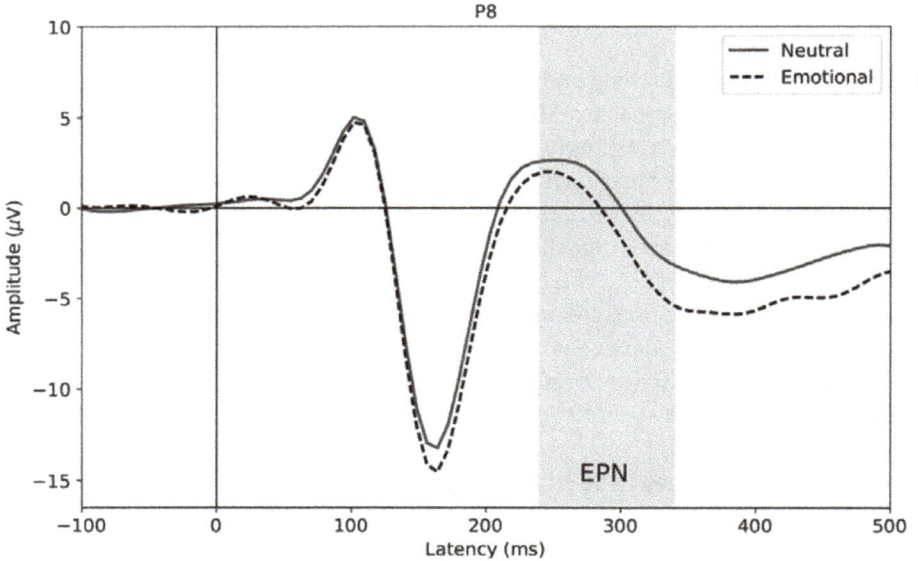

Fig. 2.3: The example of ERP waveform as presented in our previous article [37]. It presents the difference between ERPs, especially in the EPN component, evoked with neutral and emotional (happy and angry) face image stimuli.

component is known to be emotion sensitive [35, 36], which we confirmed in another study [37] (Fig. 2.3). The majority of papers on EEG emotion correlates (72 out of 130) can be found in ERP studies [29]. In standard ERP experiments, the trials have to be repeated dozens of times and averaged to enhance the signal and attenuate the noise, but there are also examples of effective online single-trial ERP classifiers [38].

2.3.2 Spectral density (frequency domain)

The spectral density of the EEG signal can be obtained using a Fourier transform. It reflects the power of brain activity in different frequency bands. Specific bands are sometimes called brain waves or neural oscillations; the most popular ones are alpha (8–12 Hz), theta (4–8 Hz), beta (13–30 Hz), and gamma (30–70 Hz) waves. The spectral power of alpha brain waves is one of the best-known markers of engagement and alertness—the lower the power in the alpha range, the higher the engagement. The power of alpha waves is also connected with discrete emotions of happiness, sadness, and fear [39]. The asymmetry of the EEG spectrum between frontal parts of different hemispheres of the brain is known as a steady correlate of valence [40]. Studies in the higher-frequency gamma band showed a significant interaction between valence and hemisphere, suggesting that the left part of the brain is involved more in positive emotions than the right hemisphere [41]. More complex emotion correlates are defined in terms of coherence between different areas of the brain; for example, the phase synchronization between frontal and right temporo-parietal regions has been connected with higher valence and arousal [42], and the coherence between prefrontal and posterior beta oscillations has been shown to increase while watching highly arousing images [43].

2.4 Introduction to machine learning

2.4.1 The concept of machine learning

Machine learning is now understood as the application of methods in the field of computer science, mathematics, and similar fields for the automatic collection of knowledge and drawing conclusions based on the provided data. Attempts to use computers for more complex tasks than just mathematical calculations took place in the 1950s, shortly after the construction of fully electronic computers. The application of statistical methods gave hope for automatic drawing conclusions from a large number of examples given to the input of algorithms. Computers were called *electronic brains*, and it was thought that in a short time they would be used in tasks such as text translation, speech recognition, and understanding and would also help to understand the functioning of the human brain. A system that fulfills such tasks was supposed to be called artificial intelligence (AI). A test, called the *Turing test*, was even proposed by Alan Turing to check if the system exhibits "intelligence" features [44]. In general, it relied on conducting a conversation in natural language and assessing its course by a judge. If the judge could not tell if he was talking with a man or a machine, it meant that the machine was intelligent. However, it turned out that the development of such a system is not easy, and the results were far from expected. In the 1970s, the initial enthusiasm dropped, and research in this field slowed down. The period of reduced interest in AI called later *AI winter* lasted until the 1990s of the twentieth century [45]. One of the reasons for failures could be modest computing capabilities of computers at that time, millions of times smaller than those currently available even in portable devices.

At present, there are programs that effectively simulate a human-made conversation and can pass the Turing test. However, the condition for recognizing a computer as "intelligent" is still shifted, and new requirements are set. Currently, the term "artificial general intelligence" is applied to a theoretical system that can take over any task that requires intelligence and cognitive skills. Such a system could, through further improvement (also self-improvement), get more skills than a human and lead to a point called *singularity*, beyond which it will not be possible to stop it and predict the development. In popular applications, the term "artificial intelligence" is used in relation to machine learning of varying degrees of sophistication.

2.4.2 The importance of data sets

As mentioned earlier, one of the reasons for failures in applying machine learning methods at the beginning of their development was the insufficient size of learning sets. Many machine learning systems are formally classifiers, i.e., systems assigning an appropriate label to a previously unknown object based on information collected by the analysis of a suitably large training set, usually already labeled.

One of the approaches to the construction of classifiers is artificial neural networks developed for decades [46]. The concept refers to a structure found in the brains of living organisms. The information is processed by a network of interconnected neurons. Neuron sums up the signals received at its inputs, scaled by the so-called weights, and then the obtained sum is converted by an activation function. This function computes the response of the neuron, its transition into an active state. The network may contain many neurons, usually organized in layers. The input data are passed to the inputs of the first layer, and the result of the classification is read from the last one.

To make a proper classification, such a network requires computing a lot of parameters—weights of connection. The determination of these weights is usually performed by numerical methods in subsequent iterations in which the error of the response generated by the network is reduced. Depending on the model used, a "feature vector" calculated with separate functions may be passed to the network input—the numbers describing selected properties of the input samples or even directly the values of the samples may be passed. In the second case, initial layers of the network are responsible for extracting features.

2.5 Automatic emotion recognition using machine learning

The visual analysis of the EEG signal is not easy even for researchers or physicians experienced in the domain. Physiological signals, especially EEG, introduce problems with noise, artifacts, and low signal-to-noise ratio. The computerized process is necessary to increase the diagnostic value of EEG. The emotion recognition is a great example of a problem that is resolvable only with the support of modern methods of machine learning. This chapter presents modern solutions for this problem, explains the process of designing emotion classifiers using machine learning, and lists state-of-the-art methods and applications.

2.5.1 Sources of the data

Three modern EEG caps from research-grade systems are presented in Fig. 2.4. Majority of works in the literature is based on these devices [29]. Besides the EEG cap, the EEG amplifier is of the greatest importance when recording high-quality data.

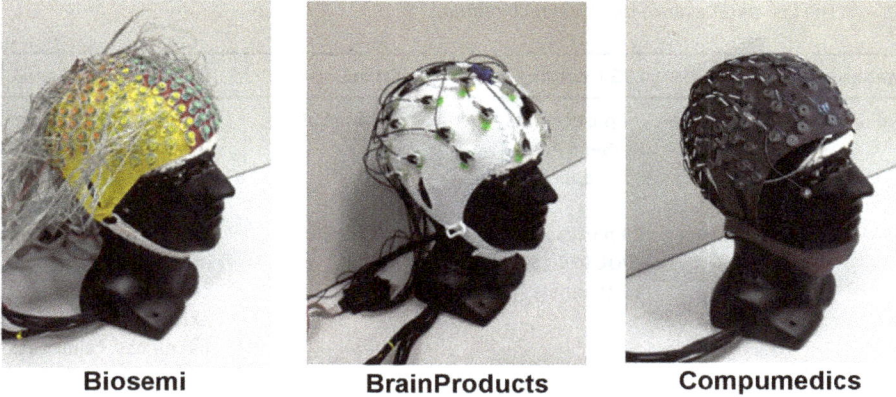

Biosemi   **BrainProducts**   **Compumedics**

Fig. 2.4: Three most popular EEG caps from research-grade EEG systems. From left to right: Biosemi ActiveTwo 128 channels (Biosemi, Amsterdam, Netherlands), BrainProducts ActiCap 32 channels (Brain Products Inc., Gilching, Germany) and Compumedics Quik-Cap 64 channels (Compumedics, Victoria, Australia).

It should provide a sampling rate of at least 256 Hz (to record a whole effective spectrum of the brain activity), the resolution at the level of nanovolts and additional channels for electrooculography or accelerometers. Because of the high cost of these systems, there is an increasing interest in using low-cost commercial EEG systems like Emotiv EPOC+ [37].

2.5.1.1 EEG data sets

There are several publicly accessible data sets for emotion recognition from EEG signals (Tab. 2.1). Arguably, the most popular one in the literature is the Database for Emotion Analysis Using Physiological Signals (DEAP) [47]. It contains EEG recordings (BioSemi ActiveTwo with 32 channels according to the 10–20 international positioning system at 512 Hz sampling frequency) from 32 participants watching 40 one-minute long music videos. Participants rated each video in terms of the levels of arousal, valence, and dominance using nine-level self-assessment manikins. Also, they rated like/dislike and familiarity of the video. The mean locations of the stimuli videos in all mentioned dimension of assessment are presented in Fig. 2.5.

Other publicly available EEG databases for emotion recognition are listed in the table below (Tab. 2.1). Majority of them use video clips as stimuli for emotion elicitation.

2.5.1.2 EEG simulators

EEG simulators, besides being the data source for algorithms testing, can be a useful tool for tutoring and teaching physicians to recognize not only emotional states but also epilepsy, pain, or depth of anesthesia of monitored patients. However, there

Tab. 2.1: The EEG databases for emotion recognition.

Database name (year)	EEG recording details	Stimuli used	Emotions model used
DEAP [47] (2012)	32 participants, BioSemi ActiveTwo, 32 channels, 512 Hz	40 video clips	Valence and arousal levels divided into four classes: HAHV, LAHV, HALV, and LALV
DREAMER [48] (2018)	23 participants, Emotiv EPOC low-cost EEG, 16 channels, 128 Hz	18 video clips	PAD model levels and nine discrete emotion classes: amusement, excitement, happiness, calmness, anger, disgust, fear, sadness, and surprise
MAHNOB-HCI [49] (2012)	27 participants, BioSemi ActiveTwo, 32 channels, 1024 Hz	20 video clips	Valence and arousal levels, nine discrete emotion classes: neutral, anxiety, amusement, sadness, joy, disgust, anger, surprise, and fear
SEED [50] (2018)	15 participants, ESI NeuroScan System, 62 channels, 1000 Hz	72 video clips	Valence and arousal levels, four discrete emotion classes: happiness, sadness, neutral, and fear
eNTERFACE06_EMOBRAIN [51] (2006)	16 participants, BioSemi ActiveTwo, 54 channels, 1024 Hz	327 images from IAPS	Three discrete emotion classes: calm, exciting positive, and exciting negative
USTC-ERVS [52] (2014, no longer available online)	28 participants, Neuroscan Synamps2, 32 channels, 500 Hz	92 video clips	Valence and arousal levels

is currently no standardized method of teaching EEG interpretation in residency programs. There are some initial works on creating software EEG simulators for teaching [53, 54], including a recent ongoing study with promising results in education [55]. Besides, there are several general-purpose EEG simulators, including the recent open-source EEG software simulator SEREEGA [56] (mainly for ERPs) and free BESA simulator. This kind of software may be integrated into virtual patient environments [57] to enhance the experience and extend the range of training scenarios.

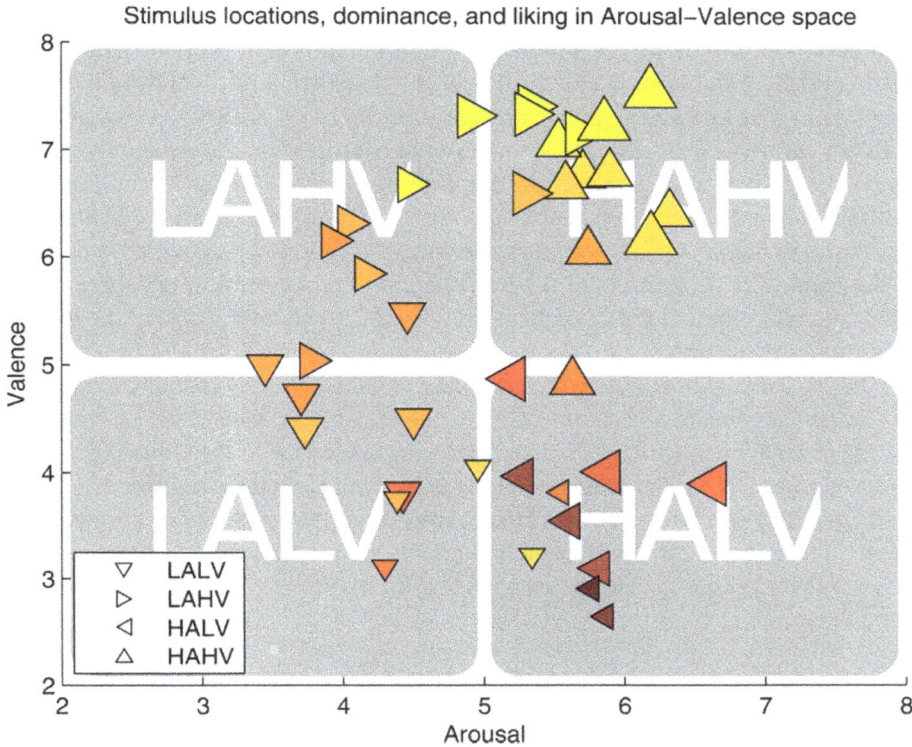

Fig. 2.5: The visualization of the DEAP database as presented by Koelstra *et al.* [47]. Triangles mark the mean locations of the stimuli on the arousal-valence plane divided into four conditions (LALV, HALV, LAHV, HAHV). Liking is encoded by color: dark red is low liking and bright yellow is high liking. Dominance is encoded by symbol size: small symbols stand for low dominance and big for high dominance.

The only commercially available hardware EEG simulator is the five-channel MiniSim 330 simulator. The recent design of hardware EEG simulator in the form of a physical phantom head is worth mentioning [58]. However, for now, hardware simulators are only used for testing EEG instruments and may never be necessary for medical training that will be based on software simulators that are easier to share, maintain, adapt, and extend.

2.5.1.3 Custom EEG experiments

The most challenging method of acquiring necessary EEG data for further analysis is to perform a new custom experiment on a group of participants. The design of such an experiment requires broad knowledge in the domain and much patience during recordings. However, it is an essential part of each research to validate the method or hypothesis on the real-world data from own experiment. In fact, each

EEG medical diagnostic procedure is an experiment that is designed to test the hypothesis that the patient is healthy. To test the hypothesis correctly using EEG, it is extremely important to strictly follow the instruction and conditions of the experiment. Our knowledge about processes in the brain is very limited, so confounding variables (extra variables that are not controlled in the experiment) may have an undefined critical effect on the brain response. The list of confounding variables is usually very long: age and gender of participants (many confirmed differences), the effect of the researcher (the way instructions are provided, presence during experiment), the time of the day, the mood and motivation of the participant, left/right handedness (if participant responds by button push), or the effects of drugs and stimulants.

The independent variable (the controlled variable) in the emotion recognition experiments is usually a class (or value in the circumplex model) of emotion that intends to be elicited using the specific stimuli. According to the thorough survey of Al-Nafjan *et al.* [29], the most frequently used stimulus type is an affective image (more than 35% of articles) before videos, music, and other modalities like games or imagination techniques. The dependent variable (the output of the experiment) in EEG experiments is defined in the selected feature space (time or frequency) as listed in chapter 2.5.2.1.

2.5.2 Methods

The process of designing any EEG automatic classifier has similar steps presented in Fig. 2.6. The differences lay mainly in the types of stimuli, extracted features, and machine learning models. This chapter is focused on presenting the overview of recently used methods as described in more detail in a few review papers [29, 31, 59, 60].

2.5.2.1 Preprocessing

The first standard step after collecting the necessary EEG data is preprocessing. Usually, it involves artifacts rejection based on excessive peak-to-peak amplitudes (over 70–100 µV), filtering using band-pass filters to remove low-frequency potential drift (under 0.5 Hz, caused i.e., by sweating) and high-frequency oscillations (over 40–70 Hz, usually containing only noise), as well as 50-Hz noise from the electric network. Frequently, the signal from each electrode is re-referenced to the average of all channels to remove common environmental artifacts; this is called *common average reference*. The independent component analysis may be used to remove external sources of noise, for example, the eyeblink or cardiac rhythm artifacts. The example of a detailed preprocessing pipeline for ERP analysis in emotion processing can be found in our previous work [37].

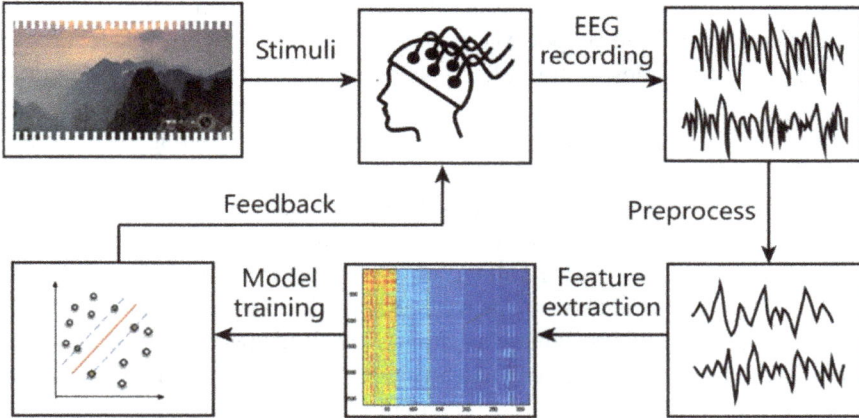

Fig. 2.6: The block diagram of a standard procedure for designing an automatic emotion recognition system, as presented by Zheng and Lu [61].

2.5.2.2 Feature extraction

The EEG data are usually high dimensional (in terms of a number of samples and number of channels in each trial), so the limited number of features should be extracted to simplify the model, speed up the training, and increase generalization. The optimal approach would be to search through all the possible EEG channels, spectral bands, and time segments for a set of features that maximize the classification score. In practice, the majority of recent automatic classification systems use properties of power spectral density bands as the main features [29, 31]. They are fast and easy to calculate and allow online classification in applications such as patients monitoring. An additional advantage in the medical context is that most physicians are familiar with these types of features. The common properties of a frequency band may be extracted as mean power, frontal asymmetry, or higher order crossing. In terms of time domain, the simple statistics of the signal like root mean square of the signal, mean, standard deviation, or entropy are usually not enough to effectively predict more emotional states. Surprisingly, considering a number of known ERP correlates of emotion, very few papers extract features from ERP waveforms. One of them is the study of Frantzidis *et al.* [62], where the amplitudes of P100, N100, P200, N200, and P300 components are used as supportive features together with frequency bands. The feature extraction step may be omitted when using deep learning methods (usually deep artificial neural networks) that select proper features as an integral part of the training procedure.

2.5.2.3 Emotion classification and estimation using machine learning

Machine learning classification (for discrete classes of emotions) and regression (for continuous emotion space) models are extensively used in the domain literature.

The most common classification method in the emotion recognition domain (like in many other domains) is the support vector machine (SVM). In short, this technique is designed to find the most representative samples that will become the "support vectors" in the feature space. The support vectors define the decision boundary (the optimal hyperplane) separating one class from another. There is also the possibility to use support vectors in the regression task when working on continuous emotion model. Another popular model in the EEG domain is the k-nearest neighbors classifier/regressor. Similarly to SVM, it is based on the comparison of the testing data to the previously provided training data. Specifically, if the majority of these k-closest training samples represent one particular class the testing sample probably also belongs to the same class. Other classifiers successfully used for emotion recognition are linear discriminant analysis and artificial neural networks. In recent years, the deep artificial neural networks have rapidly become more important because of the simplicity of use (lack of feature extraction, or sometimes even signal preprocessing steps) and prevailing results [63].

2.5.3 Results

The physicians familiar with EEG analysis are usually trained to recognize patterns of EEG changes in the time domain (seizures) and in the frequency domain (depth of anesthesia, psychiatric disorders). However, the accuracy of the diagnosis is limited by human perception, the experience of the physician, and the state of knowledge about the brain, so computerized methods can easily overperform humans. The results reported in the literature achieve levels of 82–94% for two-class (such as arousal vs. neutral or happiness vs. sadness) and 66–82% for four-class classification (such as HAHV, HALV, LALV, and LAHV classes or joy, anger, sadness, and pleasure) [31]. On the example of the DEAP data set, Li *et al.* [63] shows the comparison of accuracies using different classifiers of HAHV, HALV, LALV, and LAHV classes: 45% for the random decision forest, 63% for the kNN, 67% for the SVM, 70% for convolutional neural network, and 75% for hybrid neural network presented in the article. On the example of the eNTERFACE06_EMOBRAIN database, the best classification accuracy among calm, exciting positive, and exciting negative emotional states is achieved around 77% [64]. On the SEED data set, the emotion classification into positive, neutral, and negative classes has achieved accuracy up to 83% [65]. Presented accuracies are virtually unreachable even for human experts.

2.5.4 Applications

Automatic recognition of emotions may find, and finds, many applications. Data are not only frequently derived from the EEG but also combined with visual information (facial expressions), voice analysis, and other physiological signals like electrocardiogram or galvanic skin response. The medical applications include mainly diagnosis and monitoring of patients, and the nonmedical ones are mainly associated with brain-computer interfaces. An extensive review of EEG applications in emotion recognition from over 300 papers is presented by Al-Nafjan et al. [29].

For example, Friedrich et al. [66] described a neurofeedback game that teaches emotions for children with ASD. Children undergoing therapy were to control brain wave activity in selected bands by playing a game controlled by these waves. Studies have shown an improvement in various aspects of social interaction. Markiewcz [67] described the use of EEG measurements and feedback in the treatment of diseases as depression, autism, schizophrenia, neurosis, and Parkinson's disease.

The application of automatic emotion recognition in the effective diagnosis of Parkinson disease is presented by Yuvaraj et al. [68]. EEG signals were recorded from 20 patients with Parkinson's disease and 20 healthy participants while watching video clips. Using an SVM classifier, the samples were grouped and classified as six emotions: sadness, happiness, fear, anger, surprise, and disgust. Patients with Parkinson's disease responded less to visual stimuli. This was particularly true in the case of negative emotions.

The diagnosis of ASD in children was successfully applied using the theta coherence index, as described by Yeung et al. [69]. It is also possible to diagnose Asperger's syndrome using the task of recognizing facial expressions. Patients with Asperger's syndrome have deficiencies in the unconscious processing of coarse information—there is no N400 component. They count only on voluntary attention in recognizing emotional expression [70].

To diagnose schizophrenia in the study [71], 108 healthy and 108 schizophrenic patients observed emotional images, including sadness, fear, anger, disgust, and happiness, while ERP was recorded in conscious and unconscious conditions. The results showed that patients with schizophrenia had shorter brain activity, around 70 ms. Also, patients with schizophrenia in response to disgust had a positive pulse after 70 ms, and normal people had a negative pulse in response to fear and anger compared with happiness in the temporal-occipital regions. Significant differences between the two groups were obtained by analysis of variance (ANOVA).

In the study of depressive disorders, emotions were generated using music [72] and face images expressing the basic Ekman emotions [73]. The first study showed that patients with depression have significantly (in terms of ANOVA) more complex EEG signals in the parietal and frontal lobes compared with healthy people, and this complexity can be reduced by listening to music. In the second study, the connectivity of brain network functions was analyzed by separating coherence between brain waves. Total consistency in the gamma band has proven to be a promising indicator of depression with lower overall values for healthy people. In addition, abnormal connections were reported in patients with depression.

2.6 Summary

The connection between emotions and health is recent of high interest in the fields of medicine and psychology. The affective computing subdomain of automatic emotion recognition systems may help significantly push forward this research. The number of applications, promising results, and many open issues motivate researchers to work on this topic. However, very few papers on computational models of emotion recognition involve psychological and medical experts to validate the approach and cooperate with computer scientists. Machine learning has the potential to initiate a breakthrough in neuroscience and medical domain. The recent interest and advancements in automatic emotion recognition open new possibilities in terms of medical diagnosis and treatment. Although provided with the proper amount of good quality data, these computerized methods exceed human capabilities at a large extent. By contrast, this topic is very controversial in terms of privacy policies and recent general data protection regulation. Thus, each EEG experiment has to be accepted by the proper ethics committee and preceded by a written consent of the patient. The presented machine learning approach may be analogically applied in other physiological signals and other diagnostic fields.

2.7 Acknowledgments

This work was supported by statutory funds for young researchers of Institute of Informatics, Silesian University of Technology, Gliwice, Poland (BKM/560/RAU2/2018).

2.8 References

[1] Varsavsky A, Mareels I, Cook M. *Epileptic Seizures and the EEG: Measurement, Models, Detection and Prediction*. 1st ed. Boca Raton: CRC Press, 2010.

[2] Alotaiby TN, Alshebeili SA, Alshawi T, Ahmad I, Abd El-Samie FE. "EEG seizure detection and prediction algorithms: a survey." *EURASIP Journal on Advances in Signal Processing* 2014, no. 1 (December 2014).

[3] Marchant N, et al. "How electroencephalography serves the anesthesiologist." *Clinical EEG and Neuroscience* 45, no. 1 (January 2014): 22–32.

[4] Purdon PL, Sampson A, Pavone KJ, Brown EN. "Clinical electroencephalography for anesthesiologists: Part I." *Anesthesiology* 123, no. 4 (October 2015): 937–60.

[5] Bosl WJ, Tager-Flusberg H, Nelson CA. "EEG analytics for early detection of autism spectrum disorder: a data-driven approach." *Scientific Reports* 8, no. 1 (May 2018): 6828.

[6] Adeli H, Ghosh-Dastidar S. *Automated EEG-Based Diagnosis of Neurological Disorders: Inventing the Future of Neurology*. 1st ed. Boca Raton, FL: CRC Press, 2010.

[7] Isaac C, Januel D. "Neural correlates of cognitive improvements following cognitive remediation in schizophrenia: a systematic review of randomized trials." *Socioaffective Neuroscience and Psychology* 6, no. 1 (January 2016): 30054.

[8] Campos C, et al. "Neuroplastic changes following social cognition training in schizophrenia: a systematic review." *Neuropsychology Review* 26, no. 3 (September 2016): 310–28.

[9] Acharya UR, Sudarshan VK, Adeli H, Santhosh J, Koh JEW, Adeli A. "Computer-aided diagnosis of depression using EEG signals." *European Neurology* 73, no. 5–6 (2015): 329–36.

[10] Badrakalimuthu VR, Swamiraju R, de Waal H. "EEG in psychiatric practice: to do or not to do?" *Advances in Psychiatric Treatment* 17, no. 2 (March 2011): 114–21.

[11] Tan DEB, Tung RS, Leong WY, Than JCM. "sleep disorder detection and identification." *Procedia Engineering* 41 (2012): 289–95.

[12] Lövheim H. "A new three-dimensional model for emotions and monoamine neurotransmitters." *Medical Hypotheses* 78, no. 2 (February 2012): 341–48.

[13] Luneski A, Konstantinidis E, Bamidis PD. "Affective medicine." *Methods of Information Medicine* 49, no. 3 (January 2018): 207–18.

[14] Cohen S, Doyle WJ, Skoner DP, Rabin BS, Gwaltney JM, Jr. "Social ties and susceptibility to the common cold." *JAMA* 277, no. 24 (June 1997): 1940–4.

[15] Glaser R, Pearl DK, Kiecolt-Glaser JK, Malarkey WB. "Plasma cortisol levels and reactivation of latent Epstein-Barr virus in response to examination stress." *Psychoneuroendocrinology* 19, no. 8 (January 1994): 765–72.

[16] Picard RW. *Affective Computing*. Cambridge, MA: MIT Press, 1997.

[17] Panksepp J. *Affective Neuroscience: The Foundations of Human and Animal Emotions*. New York, NY: Oxford University Press, 1998.

[18] Ekman P. "An argument for basic emotions." *Cognition and Emotion* 6, no. 3–4 (May 1992): 169–200.

[19] Russell JA. "Core affect and the psychological construction of emotion." *Psychological Review* 110, no. 1 (2003): 145–72.

[20] Plutchik R. "The Nature of emotions: human emotions have deep evolutionary roots, a fact that may explain their complexity and provide tools for clinical practice." *American Scientist* 89, no. 4 (2001): 344–50.

[21] Cowen AS, Keltner D. "Self-report captures 27 distinct categories of emotion bridged by continuous gradients." *Proceedings of the National Academy of Sciences* 114, no. 38 (September 2017): E7900–9.

[22] Mehrabian A, Russell JA. *An approach to environmental psychology*. Cambridge, MA: The MIT Press, 1974.

[23] Russell JA, Mehrabian A. "Evidence for a three-factor theory of emotions." *Journal of Research in Personality* 11, no. 3 (September 1977): 273–94.

[24] Bakker I, van der Voordt T, Vink P, de Boon J. "Pleasure, arousal, dominance: Mehrabian and Russell revisited." *Current Psychology* 33, no. 3 (September 2014): 405–21.

[25] Russell JA, Lewicka M, Niit T. "A cross-cultural study of a circumplex model of affect." *Journal of Personality and Social Psychology* 57, no. 5 (1989): 848–56.

[26] Landowska A. "Towards new mappings between emotion representation models." *Applied Sciences* 8, no. 2 (2018): 274.

[27] Lindquist KA, Barrett LF. "A functional architecture of the human brain: emerging insights from the science of emotion." *Trends in Cognitive Sciences* 16, no. 11 (November 2012): 533–40.

[28] Wyczesany M, Ligeza TS. "Towards a constructionist approach to emotions: verification of the three-dimensional model of affect with EEG-independent component analysis." *Experimental Brain Research* 233, no. 3 (March 2015): 723–33.

[29] Al-Nafjan A, Hosny M, Al-Ohali Y, Al-Wabil A. "Review and classification of emotion recognition based on EEG brain-computer interface system research: a systematic review." *Applied Sciences* 7, no. 12 (2017).

32 —— 2 Machine learning approach to automatic recognition of emotions

[30] Bradley MM, Lang PJ. "The International Affective Picture System (IAPS) in the study of emotion and attention." In *Handbook of Emotion Elicitation and Assessment*, pp. 29–46. New York, NY: Oxford University Press, 2007.

[31] Kim MK, Kim M, Oh E, Kim SP. "A review on the computational methods for emotional state estimation from the human EEG." *Computational and Mathematical Methods in Medicine* 2013 (2013): 1–13.

[32] Olofsson JK, Nordin S, Sequeira H, Polich J. "Affective picture processing: an integrative review of ERP findings." *Biological Psychology* 77, no. 3 (March 2008): 247–65.

[33] Lithari C, et al. "Are females more responsive to emotional stimuli? A neurophysiological study across arousal and valence dimensions." *Brain Topography* 23, no. 1 (March 2010): 27–40.

[34] Rozenkrants B, Polich J. "Affective ERP processing in a visual oddball task: arousal, valence, and gender." *Clinical Neurophysiology* 119, no. 10 (October 2008): 2260–5.

[35] Eimer M, Holmes A. "Event-related brain potential correlates of emotional face processing." *Neuropsychologia* 45, no. 1 (January 2007): 15–31.

[36] Wronka E, Walentowska W. "Attention modulates emotional expression processing." *Psychophysiology* 48, no. 8 (August 2011): 1047–56.

[37] Kotowski K, Stapor K, Leski J, Kotas M. "Validation of Emotiv EPOC+ for extracting ERP correlates of emotional face processing." *Biocybernetics and Biomedical Engineering* 38, no. 4 (January 2018): 773–81.

[38] Blankertz B, Lemm S, Treder M, Haufe S, Müller KR. "Single-trial analysis and classification of ERP components—a tutorial." *NeuroImage* 56, no. 2 (May 2011): 814–25.

[39] Balconi M, Lucchiari C. "EEG correlates (event-related desynchronization) of emotional face elaboration: a temporal analysis." *Neuroscience Letters* 392, no. 1 (January 2006): 118–23.

[40] Balconi M, Mazza G. "Brain oscillations and BIS/BAS (behavioral inhibition/activation system) effects on processing masked emotional cues: ERS/ERD and coherence measures of alpha band." *International Journal of Psychophysiology* 74, no. 2 (November 2009): 158–65.

[41] Müller MM, Keil A, Gruber T, Elbert T. "Processing of affective pictures modulates right-hemispheric gamma band EEG activity." *Clinical Neurophysiology* 110, no. 11 (November 1999): 1913–20.

[42] Wyczesany M, Grzybowski S, Barry R, Kaiser J, Coenen AM, Potoczek A. "Covariation of EEG synchronization and emotional state as modified by anxiolytics." *Journal of Clinical Neurophysiology* 28, no. 3 (June 2011): 289–96.

[43] Miskovic V, Schmidt LA. "Cross-regional cortical synchronization during affective image viewing." *Brain Research* 1362 (November 2010): 102–11.

[44] Turing AM. "Computing machinery and intelligence." In *Parsing the Turing Test*, pp. 23–65. Springer, 2009.

[45] Hendler J. "Avoiding another AI winter." *IEEE Intelligent Systems* 23, no. 2 (March 2008): 2–4.

[46] Macukow B. "Neural networks—state of art, brief history, basic models and architecture." In *Computer Information Systems and Industrial Management*, pp. 3–14, 2016.

[47] Koelstra S, et al. "DEAP: a database for emotion analysis; using physiological signals." *IEEE Transactions on Affective Computing* 3, no. 1 (January 2012): 18–31.

[48] Katsigiannis S, Ramzan N. "DREAMER: a database for emotion recognition through EEG and ECG signals from wireless low-cost off-the-shelf devices." *IEEE Journal of Biomedical and Health Informatics* 22, no. 1 (January 2018): 98–107.

[49] Soleymani M, Lichtenauer J, Pun T, Pantic M. "A multimodal database for affect recognition and implicit tagging." *IEEE Transactions on Affective Computing* 3, no. 1 (January 2012): 42–55.

[50] Zheng W, Liu W, Lu Y, Lu B, Cichocki A. "EmotionMeter: a multimodal framework for recognizing human emotions." *IEEE Transactions on Cybernetics* (2018): 1–13.

[51] Savran A, et al. "Emotion detection in the loop from brain signals and facial images." In *Proceedings of the eNTERFACE 2006 Workshop*, 2006.

[52] Wang S, Zhu Y, Wu G, Ji Q. "Hybrid video emotional tagging using users' EEG and video content." *Multimedia Tools and Applications* 72, no. 2 (September 2014): 1257–83.

[53] Mayorov O. "Virtual training simulator—designer of EEG signals for tutoring students and doctors to methods of quantitative EEG analysis (qEEG)." Presented at the Medical Infobahn for Europe 2000, 2000, vol. 77, pp. 573–7.

[54] Morita K, Shiraishi Y, Sato S. "Making EEG output on human simulator." In *IEEE International Workshop on Biomedical Circuits and Systems, 2004*, pp. S3/6–12. 2004.

[55] Hubert M, Cios J, Cavalcanti M, Khurma A. "An effective tool for teaching EEG interpretation to residents and medical students (P4.5-019)." *Neurology* 92, no. 15 Supplement (April 2019).

[56] Krol LR, Pawlitzki J, Lotte F, Gramann K, Zander TO. "SEREEGA: simulating event-related EEG activity." *Journal of Neuroscience Methods* 309 (November 2018): 13–24.

[57] Kononowicz AA, Hege I. "The world of virtual patients." In *Simulations in Medicine: Pre-clinical and Clinical Applications*, pp. 121–38. Berlin, Boston: De Gruyter, 2015.

[58] Oliveira AS, Schlink BR, Hairston WD, König P, Ferris DP. "Induction and separation of motion artifacts in EEG data using a mobile phantom head device." *Journal of Neural Engineering* 13, no. 3 (May 2016).

[59] Zangeneh Soroush M, Maghooli K, Setarehdan SK, Motie Nasrabadi A. "A review on EEG signals based emotion recognition." *International Clinical Neuroscience Journal* 4, no. 4 (October 2017): 118–29.

[60] Alarcao SM, Fonseca MJ. "Emotions recognition using EEG signals: a survey." *IEEE Transactions on Affective Computing* 10 (2017): 374–93.

[61] Wei-Long Zheng, Bao-Liang Lu. "Investigating critical frequency bands and channels for EEG-based emotion recognition with deep neural networks." *IEEE Transactions on Autonomous Mental Development* 7, no. 3 (September 2015): 162–75.

[62] Frantzidis CA, Bratsas C, Papadelis CL, Konstantinidis E, Pappas C, Bamidis PD. "Toward emotion aware computing: an integrated approach using multichannel neurophysiological recordings and affective visual stimuli." *IEEE Transactions on Information Technology in Biomedicine* 14, no. 3 (May 2010): 589–97.

[63] Li Y, Huang J, Zhou H, Zhong N. "Human emotion recognition with electroencephalographic multidimensional features by hybrid deep neural networks." *Applied Sciences* 7, no. 10 (October 2017): 1060.

[64] Khalili Z, Moradi MH. "Emotion recognition system using brain and peripheral signals: using correlation dimension to improve the results of EEG." In *2009 International Joint Conference on Neural Networks*, pp. 1571–5, 2009.

[65] Li X, Song D, Zhang P, Zhang Y, Hou Y, Hu B. "Exploring EEG features in cross-subject emotion recognition." *Frontiers in Neuroscience* 12 (March 2018): 162.

[66] Friedrich EVC, et al. "An effective neurofeedback intervention to improve social interactions in children with autism spectrum disorder." *Journal of Autism and Developmental Disorders* 45, no. 12 (December 2015): 4084–100.

[67] Markiewcz R. "The use of EEG biofeedback/neurofeedback in psychiatric rehabilitation." *Psychiatria Polska* 51, no. 6 (December 2017): 1095–106.

[68] Yuvaraj R, et al. "Detection of emotions in Parkinson's disease using higher order spectral features from brain's electrical activity." *Biomedical Signal Processing and Control* 14 (November 2014): 108–16.

[69] Yeung MK, Han YMY, Sze SL, Chan AS. "Altered right frontal cortical connectivity during facial emotion recognition in children with autism spectrum disorders." *Research in Autism Spectrum Disorders* 8, no. 11 (November 2014): 1567–77.

[70] Tseng YL, Yang HH, Savostyanov AN, Chien VSC, Liou M. "Voluntary attention in Asperger's syndrome: brain electrical oscillation and phase-synchronization during facial emotion recognition." *Research in Autism Spectrum Disorders* 13–14 (May 2015): 32–51.

[71] Brennan AM, Harris AWF, Williams LM. "Neural processing of facial expressions of emotion in first onset psychosis." *Psychiatry Research* 219, no. 3 (November 2014): 477–85.

[72] Akdemir Akar S, Kara S, Agambayev S, Bilgiç V. "Nonlinear analysis of EEGs of patients with major depression during different emotional states." *Computers in Biology and Medicine* 67 (December 2015): 49–60.

[73] Li Y, Cao D, Wei L, Tang Y, Wang J. "Abnormal functional connectivity of EEG gamma band in patients with depression during emotional face processing." *Clinical Neurophysiology* 126, no. 11 (November 2015): 2078–89.

Grzegorz Marcin Wójcik

3 Selected methods of quantitative analysis in electroencephalography

3.1 Introduction

Electroencephalography (EEG) has been known for about 100 years and covers the techniques used for detecting and recording the electrical activity of the brain cortex. It is hard to state who invented the EEG; however, most often three researchers are mentioned in the literature: Richard Caton, Hans Berger, and Adolf Abraham Beck [1, 2].

Richard Caton (1842–1926) was a physician, a physiologist, and Lord Mayor of Liverpool, where he moved from Edinburgh in the late sixties of the nineteenth century and lived there until the end of his life. Caton used galvanometer to detect the electrical activity of the rabbit's, dog's, and monkey's brains. He put the electrodes directly on the surface of the cortex or on the skull, which can be treated as the beginning of EEG [1–3].

Caton's research was noted by Hans Berger (1873–1941): "Caton has already published experiments on the brains of dogs and apes in which bare unipolar electrodes were placed either on the cerebral cortex or on the skull surface. The currents were measured by a sensitive galvanometer. There were found distinct variations in current which increased during sleep and with the onset of death strengthened. After death they became weaker and then completely disappeared" [1, 4]. Initially, this German psychiatrist studied mathematics, and after the accident in the cavalry, where he was drafted for 1 year, he resigned of becoming an astronomer and finally became a medical doctor at the University of Jena. He was the first to observe the alpha waves (see Fig. 3.1), originally called Berger rhythms, and is recognized as the father of EEG by many historians of neuroscience. He suffered from clinical depression and committed suicide by hanging himself in his clinic in 1941 [1].

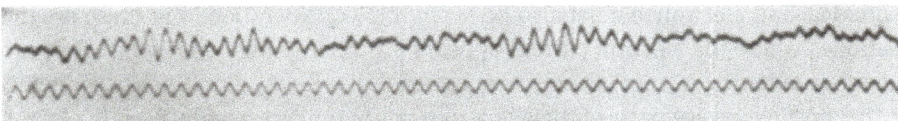

Fig. 3.1: Recording of alpha waves from the Berger's works in 1929 [4].

Adolph Abraham Beck (1863–1942) was a Polish professor of physiology at Jagiellonian University in Cracow where he studied medicine and attracted great attention in Western Europe by publishing in 1890–1891 [5, 6]. Since that time, he has been regarded as one of the pioneers of EEG. Unfortunately, he also committed suicide during the war (1942) in Janowska concentration camp in Lwów.

EEG is a noninvasive, relatively cheap and effective method in the diagnosis of epilepsy, widely applied in clinics and other medical institutions for years. However, in the last two decades, its renaissance was observed as some new algorithms were proposed making it possible to model the cortex electrical activity in time and space, sometimes with possibility of looking deeper into the brain subcortical structures.

This chapter presents the fundamental methods of quantitative EEG (qEEG) with its typical applications accompanied by useful software review and some tips and tricks that may improve the quality of the undertaken research.

3.2 EEG technology and resting state

The electrical activity of the brain cortex is recorded using a set of electrodes and amplifiers. Amplifiers transmit the registered activity most often to the computer where the signal is recorded on the hard disk. The recorded signal can be then cleaned, preprocessed, and postprocessed without the necessity of the patient's presence in the lab.

Before discussing technology, it is necessary to understand how long and hard way the signal must go through before it can be recorded. The cortex is composed of tens of billions of neural cells called neurons. Each neuron has its base potential equal to approximately −70 mV and reaching +40 mV during excitations. It must be remembered that the current in the brain has ionic character, as the potential on neural cells is a result of potassium, sodium, and chloride ions dynamics across the membrane. Considering the typical shape of the head and the size of the brain that is a bit smaller than the size of the head, one can imagine the size of the cortex that covers the subcortical areas of the brain. Next, when electrodes are placed on the head, the signal registered by one electrode is assumed to come from millions of neurons. To be registered, the electrical potential must be probed deeply through the hair, some dirt and fat on the scalp, the scalp itself, the skull, some blood, meninges, and cerebrospinal fluid. The appropriate contact (impedance) between scalp, metal electrodes, and electrolyte must also be taken into consideration, and these are the electrodes where the electron current appears for the first time and in fact they are converters of ionic current to the electron current. That is why amplifiers used in EEG are the most expensive parts of the whole system. Amplifiers usually used in clinical practice consist of 16–24 electrodes. There are also amplifiers with a smaller number of electrodes, sometimes even two-electrode amplifiers, used for game industry or simple experiments [7], including neurofeedback techniques [8] or brain-computer interfaces. The most advanced EEG labs are equipped with the so-called dense array amplifiers with 256 [9] or very rarely 512 operating electrodes. To provide appropriate impedance between the electrode and the scalp, different substances are used to moisture the electrode—from the gel-based substances to electrolyte solution filling up the sponge in the electrode socket. The best EEG labs are also equipped with eye trackers that allow eliminating eye blink artifacts or saccadic eye movements and photogrammetry stations owing to which it is possible to place particular electrodes on the later-generated model of the brain.

The simplest EEG experiment is called the resting state. During the experiment, the subject is sitting, often with closed eyes, doing nothing, not moving. The activity of the brain is then registered for several minutes, and the laboratory staff can then observe the changes of activity during the resting state. It is the resting state where, for example, epilepsy can be observed. As a result, we obtain the table of numbers, like a typical spreadsheet, with the number of columns equal the number of electrodes and one additional column in which the time is registered. The number of rows in the table depends on the probing frequency and the length of the experiment. The best amplifiers allow to record the signal with a 1,000-Hz probing frequency. The frequency usually is set to 250 Hz, which means that 250 rows are added to the table for each second of the experiment. This makes the EEG far ahead of all competitors, including fMRI, in the temporal resolution category.

In Fig. 3.2, the Laboratory of EEG in the Chair of Neuroinformatics and Biomedical Engineering (CoNaBI),[1] Maria Curie-Sklodowska University in Lublin, Poland,

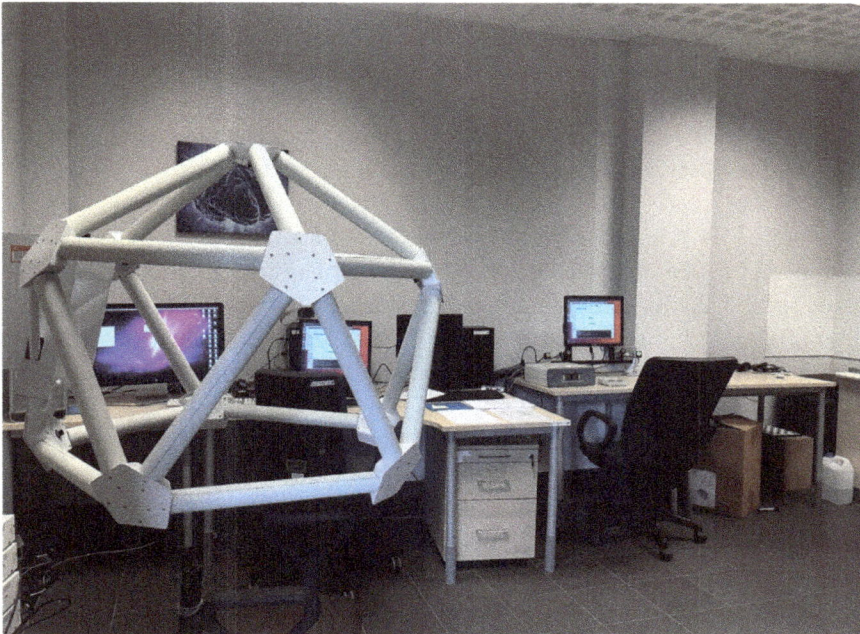

Fig. 3.2: Laboratory of EEG in the Chair of Neuroinformatics and Biomedical Engineering (CoNaBI).

---

[1] Chair of Neuroinformatics and Biomedical Engineering, Maria Curie-Sklodowska University in Lublin, ul. Akademicka 9, 20-033 Lublin, Poland. E-mail: gmwojcik@live.umcs.lublin.pl.

is presented. It is equipped with the dense array amplifier able to record the brain electrical activity with 500-Hz frequency through 256 channel HydroCel GSN 130 Geodesic Sensor Nets.

The laboratory is a complete and compatible system provided by electrical geodesic systems (EGI).[2] In addition, the geodesic photogrammetry system (GPS) was used, which makes a model of subject brain based on its calculated size, proportion, and shape, owing to 11 cameras placed in its corners, and then puts all computed activity results on this model with very good accuracy. The amplifier works with the Net Station 4.5.4 software, GPS under the control of the Net Local 1.00.00, and Geo-Source 2.0. Gaze calibration, eye blinks, and saccades elimination are obtained, owing to the application of eye tracking system operated by SmartEye 5.9.7. The event-related potential (ERP) experiments are designed in the PST e-Prime 2.0.8.90 environment.

3.3 EEG rhythms and power spectrum

However, current EEG is not only looking at the wormlike plots of the registered potentials. The real power of technology manifests itself when cortical activity is treated in a quantitative way. Probably the oldest quantitative method of EEG is the application of Fourier transforms to the signal. The power spectrum allows to find the dominant rhythms, sometimes called EEG bands, as it becomes possible to see how much amount of sine waves with particular frequencies contribute to the whole signal. A nice metaphor comes to my mind as an example—the neurons in the brain cortex tend to play music like crickets in the meadow, and they play synchronically. Thus, the rhythm observed in the cortex is characteristic of its large part, not only for the single electrode.

There are six most important EEG rhythms: δ, delta band (less than 4 Hz) often observed in babies; θ, theta (4–7 Hz)—greater in young children; α, alpha (8–15 Hz)—associated with relaxation, closed eyes, and meditation; β, beta (16–31 Hz)—in stress or active thinking; γ, gamma (more than 31 Hz)—when short-term memory is engaged and during cross stimulation; sometimes μ, mu (8–12 Hz)—in motor neurons in the resting state [10].

The question that should be asked right now is about the length of the signal that should be taken to the Fourier transforms. Obviously, there is not much sense in finding the dominant frequency in the whole signal, lasting, for example, for an hour as this may change in time. The answer depends on the conducted experiment. Sometimes just a few seconds is enough, and in another case, this may be one minute. One thing is certain—spectral analysis is still useful in the quantitative research of cortical electrical activity.

---

2 Electrical Geodesic Systems, Inc., 500 East 4th Ave. Suite 200, Eugene, OR 97401, USA.

3.4 Event-related potentials

Another method with the fundamental applications in qEEG is the observation of ERPs. Quite often, when we tell someone who is not familiar with neuroscience about the EEG, the question whether it is possible to see the manifestation of a luxury car or a beautiful woman in the cortical activity is asked. Unfortunately, it is not possible to notice this in a single EEG trial. However, if such stimuli were shown more than once, it would probably be possible to get a hold of something. Such an approach to the experiment is called ERP [11]. Some events evoke some reactions in the brain, and when the whole process is treated statistically, there will appear measurable curves, indicating characteristic response to the stimuli.

Probably the most famous ERP experiment is the so-called P300. During the experimental trial, the subjects are asked to press buttons whenever they can see a cross on the computer screen. There are only two objects that can be shown on the black screen of the computer: a white circle (80% of stimuli) and a white cross (20% of stimuli). The circles are called standards, whereas the crosses are called targets. All symbols are shown 400 times in total. The subject expects to see the cross each time the stimulus is shown. He or she hunts for targets. Unfortunately, in 80% of cases, the subject is disappointed. However, when the target stimulus appears—the button is pressed. Actually, they do not need to press anything. We can tell what they see based only on their cortical activity owing to the ERP appearing in their brains. To get the ERP, the signal must be averaged in some set time intervals, for example, 200 ms before the stimulus and 400 ms after that. The averaged signal looks completely different from the typical EEG recording, but the extrema of the function show the appearance of the stimuli and cortical reaction to such stimulation. Note that this must be repeated many times because only the noise will be observed in single recording.

There is a variety of different ERPs appearing on different parts on the scalp, depending on the stimuli. Thus, there are visual ERPs, auditory ERPs, language-related responses, decision making–related responses, or even ERPs appearing during face recognition [11]. Numerous books have been written about the ERP, among the most worth reading is by Luck [11]. One thing is certain—it is hard to imagine current experimental psychology using EEG without ERP. We have some experience in doing ERPs in patients with psychiatric disorders, and such an approach may be useful in finding psychiatric disorder biomarkers in the EEG signal, making psychiatry more "quantitative" and experimental [12, 13].

3.5 Dipole source modeling

It has been already pointed out that in the category of temporal resolution, the EEG is much better than any other technique, especially fMRI. However, when considering the spatial resolution, it is relatively poor. That is why some algorithms have been proposed to solve this problem, and they are generally called source localization methods. Owing to them, it is possible to put EEG-based and calculated activity of a particular region of the brain on the brain model and get the resolution similar to that obtained from the computed tomography (CT). This is very important as for the first time in this chapter, the set of time series with the number of elements equal to the number of electrodes will not be discussed, but the topographic map of the brain cortex placed on the brain model and calculated from the data present in that time series will be considered.

The origin of the dipoles in the brain is strictly connected with the anatomical structure of the cortex. The electrical activity that can be registered using the EEG amplifiers comes mainly from the so-called pyramidal cells. The current flows perpendicular to the surface of the cortex because such is the alignment of the neural columns, and the electrical current coming from the dendritic trees almost totally cancels as their orientation is rotational and parallel to the cortex. Intercortical current vectors sum linearly, and the areas of about 3 cm can be very effectively modeled by a single electrical dipole. The more electrodes, the better spatial resolution is obtained. It should be remembered that the potential we measure does not come directly from the neurons that are the closest to the electrode [10, 14].

To generate the brain model with dipoles responsible for the EEG activity measured on the scalp, one must solve the inverse problem using the Laplace and the Poisson electric field equations. However, there is no space in this book to discuss it in detail. Moreover, the good news is that there are a lot of software solutions that allow treating the collected EEG signal so that the dipole source modeling (DSM) is conducted without the knowledge of highly complicated methods of applied mathematics and theoretical physics. Then the dipoles calculated from the EEG signal can be put on the standard model of the brain or when the lab is well equipped—on the real model of the subject's brain generated by means of the photogrammetry station. A lot of research in neurophysiology has been carried out using the DSM technique as the dynamics of the dipoles can shed some light on the problem impossible to be noticed when looking only at pure EEG [10, 14].

3.6 Source localization LORETA/sLORETA

One of the best-known algorithms originating from the idea of source localization is the low-resolution brain electromagnetic tomography (LORETA) and its standardized version sLORETA. Proposed by Pasqual-Marqui in 2006, it is characterized by many modifications that can be useful in some special cases of analysis [15, 16]. Based on the EEG inversed problem, these methods allow to calculate and then visualize the activity of the whole brain in the three-dimensional model consisting of voxels put on the Talairach atlas. In contrast to the DSM, we do not get the current dipoles but the map of the points of interests with calculated activity in nanoamperes and the time in which that activity occurred. We have experience in applying sLORETA for the analysis of the EEG signals in both healthy and disordered subjects in the ERP experiments [12, 13]. This method allowed us to indicate the most active Brodmann areas (BAs) on the brain cortex and in some subcortical areas like amygdala. Our findings come along with those findings of some MRI/fMRI experiments, which in some way prove the effectiveness of such an approach [12, 13].

Remembering that the electric current is defined as the electric charge flow in time, it is possible to integrate the current over time and obtain the mean electric charge flowing through the particular brain area. In the study of Wojcik et al. [12], we defined such a new measure adding some value to qEEG as it may be important whether the increased activity of the selected area lasted in time or not.

The expression of each BA through which the electric current is flowing is as follows:

$$I(\text{BA},\ t,\ \tau,\ |\psi\rangle) = \frac{\partial q(\text{BA},\ t,\ \tau,\ |\psi\rangle)}{\partial t}, \tag{1}$$

where $q(\text{BA},\ t,\ \tau,\ |\psi\rangle)$ indicates the electric current accumulated in a given period of time with the stimulation in τ. It is sure to depend on a group of psychophysiological parameters whose representation is the vector $|\psi\rangle$. ι (Iota), which is a new observable, can be termed as the electric charge flowing through the BA obtained by the following integral:

$$\forall\ \text{BA}\ :\ \iota = q(\text{BA},\ t,\ \tau,\ |\psi\rangle) = \int_{\tau+t_2}^{\tau+t_1} I(\text{BA},\ t,\ \tau,\ |\psi\rangle)\mathrm{d}t, \tag{2}$$

in the range from t_1 before and t_2 after the stimulation in τ [12].

It is crucial to note that there are still common beliefs that it is impossible to record the EEG activity from the subcortical areas, but these are wrong beliefs. Indeed, subcortical structures produce smaller scalp EEG signals. This is due to the fact that they are farther from the head surface than the cortical structures. To make matters worse, subcortical neurons can have a closed-field geometry that further weakens the observed distant fields and subcortical structures are surrounded by the cortical mantle [17]. Thus, measurements of activity in deep brain structures can be potentially explained by a surrogate distribution of currents on the cortex. That is why it can be very difficult to measure subcortical activity when cortical activity takes place at the same time [17]. However, owing to the source localization and algorithms like sLORETA—this subcortical activity can be simulated with very good accuracy, which is extensively used to understand the activity patterns appearing on the cortex while performing cognitive tasks. This can lead, as we hope, to finding some biomarkers, for example, in decision-making processes or selected psychiatric disorders on which our research is focused [12, 13].

3.7 Principal component analysis

In the zoo of quantitative methods used in EEG, the statistical methods seem to be very interesting. One of them is principal component analysis (PCA), which is used in many areas that are far away from neuroscience. PCA applies orthogonal transformations expressed by matrix operations to reduce the amount of data. Among other reasons, the PCA is often chosen to shorten the time of computations without loss of crucial information present in the system [10, 18].

During the EEG procedure, a huge data set A is obtained, and the main idea of the PCA method is to reduce the dimension of such a multidimensional data set A of variables depending on each other [10]. This can be achieved by transforming data set A into another data set B with uncorrelated elements called principal components. The elements of data set B are not correlated and often orthogonal. In data set B, the data are arranged in such a way so that the first few sum up to most of the variation present in data set A [10]. In other words, the PCA method allows to reduce the amount of information in the EEG signal by removing some less important components originating from artifacts or another noise and keeping the most important components responsible for the dynamics of the whole system.

In the aspect of ERP experiments, this method is responsible for the decomposition of the ERP curve into the component-related curves that sum up to the original one.

In the applied computational neuroscience, owing to the PCA methods, it was possible to find useful topographies and effects of interest in a wide range of experiments and neurophysiological research [10, 18].

3.8 Independent component analysis

Imagine an orchestra assembling of no more than 256 musicians playing different instruments in the concert hall. Now imagine 256 microphones recording the concert. The position of the microphones does not change during the recording time. After the concert, one obtains 256 recordings in 256 sound files. They are very similar, though quite different. The difference depends, for example, on the distance of a particular microphone from the given instrument. Try to find the position of each instrument of the orchestra in the concert hall and separate the music it plays to put it in a new sound file. In addition, the sum of all the separated sound files should give the whole concert.

Such a metaphor exemplifies the other useful qEEG method called independent component analysis (ICA). The assumption of that method is to separate the EEG signal in such a way so that it is possible to express it as a sum of temporarily independent and spatially fixed components. Contrary to the PCA, these components do not have to be orthogonal [10, 19].

Similar to the PCA, the EEG signal is treated as the huge data set. In the signal registered by one electrode, there can be many artifacts, and the influence of different brain regions placed under other electrodes can be observed. This means that one electrode does not necessarily record strictly the activity of the group of millions of neurons placed exactly under that but under ideal conditions from the whole brain.

If one wants to remove the artifacts from the signal, he should definitely try to use the ICA. ICA application also makes it possible to topographically place the origin of cortical activity registered by the electrode.

The ICA is regarded to be a blind source separation (BSS)-type algorithm. It is based on the theory of central limit according to which when the random variable is characterized by a normal distribution (recording of a single electrode), it is regarded to be a "mixture" of independent random variables (in this case, signals that are independent). The sources making up the recoded signal are assumed to be statistically independent of each other, which is the algorithm base. This results in the negative aspect of the algorithm as the effect of ICA is the minimalization of the Gaussian distribution as far as the values are disseminated. Thus, a distribution close to normal of more than one primary signal gives an ambiguous result [10, 19].

The algorithm has an unknown number of steps and is both time and power consuming. The length of computation depends on the length of the signal. The main disadvantage of the ICA is that even if it is possible to separate independent component signal frequency, it is not possible to calculate their amplitude, which is typical of BSS algorithms.

The EEG manufacturers do not often add ICA to their software solutions. That is why in many cases, the ICA must be implemented by the researcher to satisfy his or her needs and expectations.

We have experience in ICA programming. As it was mentioned above, the computations are time consuming. We proposed some methods of the ICA parallelization and tested them on different architectures [20–22]. To get satisfactory results, one ought to consider decomposition on the supercomputers or apply at least the CUDA methodology.

3.9 Software reviews

3.9.1 OpenSesame

During the design phase of each experiment, it is obligatory to choose the software that will be used to present the stimuli to the subject. There is a wide range of software solutions for the ERP experiment design; among others, the OpenSesame[3] is

---

3 OpenSesame: https://osdoc.cogsci.nl.

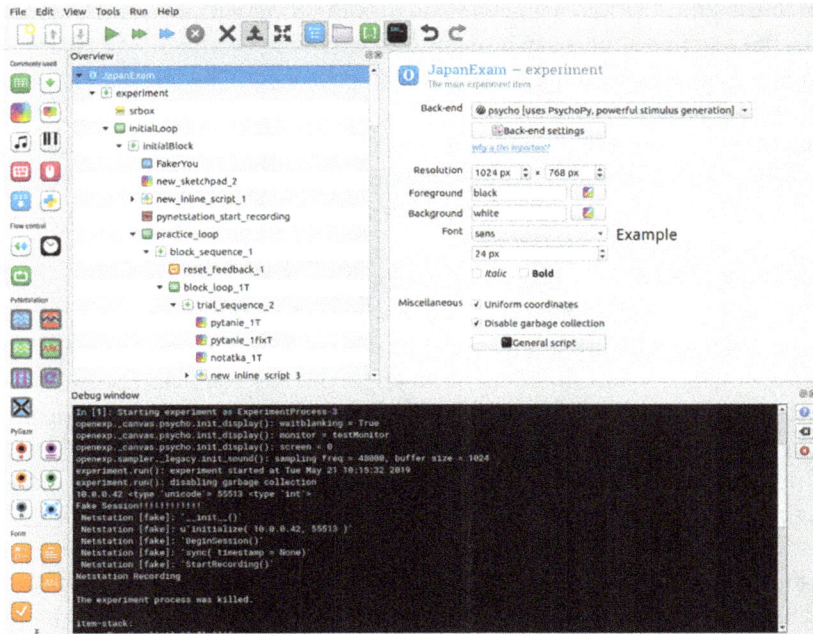

Fig. 3.3: OpenSesame interface. It allows the user to design experiments in many stimulation ways as sound or visual. Experiment can be controlled and run using the power Python scripting language. The signal can be tagged during the experiment, which makes it suitable for future postprocessing.

often chosen by experimentalists owing to its elastic interface, making it possible to present a wide range of stimuli and tag the recorded signal in the required way. It is free, available for the most popular platforms (Linux, MacOS, Windows, and even Android—only runtime), and compatible with most devices that can be found in the EEG labs like amplifiers and other EEG equipment, eye tracking systems, and response pads. The greatest power of the OpenSesame manifests itself due to the Python interface. One can design experiments with flexibility and practically an infinite range of solutions available in the Python programming language. The interface of the OpenSesame is presented in Fig. 3.3. In the case of problems, the user is also supported by the community forum, which can be useful for the researchers beginning the EEG adventure.

3.9.2 Net Station

When the experiment is designed, it must be conducted in the EEG laboratory, and signal recording is the most important phase of the experiment. There are so many possible obstacles that may make the proper recording impossible. Unfortunately, there is no space in this chapter to mention all of them. Obviously, the electromagnetic noise is the most common. Not always is it possible to use Faraday's cage due to the fact that it is huge and quite expensive. However, researchers must try to find the most electromagnetically friendly room and often the time of the day in the reality of the building in which the laboratory is situated. There may also be problems originating from the long hair of the subjects or the gender as women tend to have periodically changing electric activity of the brain. When all conditions are satisfied, and the impedance between the scalp and the electrodes is appropriate, one can start the signal recording.

The software used to record the signal and integrate it with the stimuli systems is usually provided by the amplifier manufacturer. However, it can also be developed from the scratch in which we have some experience [7, 8]. The software used in our EGI system is Net Station.[4] With its hundreds of functionalities, it allows to design the experiments from the very low-level stage, such as selecting the cable connections of all devices used in the experiment, through the multichannel recording with up to 1,000-Hz probing frequency, to the artifact elimination, such as saccadic eye movements or eye blinks. The recorded signal can be preprocessed by the Net Station and postprocessed later, and the data can be exported to many most common data formats to be transformed in any way.

The interface of Net Station is presented in Fig. 3.4. The other amplifiers are equipped with different software. It is no use to describe all of them. However, there is

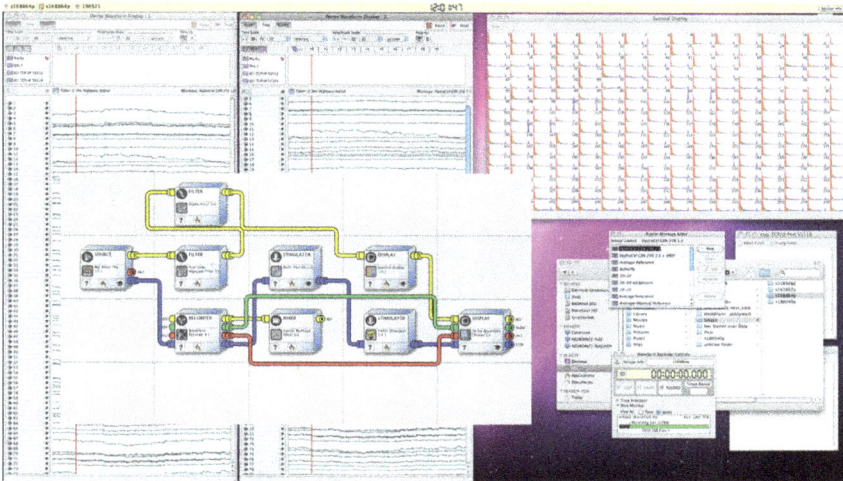

Fig. 3.4: The interface of the Net Station experiment control system. One can observe the raw signal windows as well as the online Fourier analysis (in the background). It is also possible to design particular modules and connections to prepare the most appropriate experiment setup.

---

4 Net Station Software for Clinical Use: https://www.egi.com/clinical-division/net-station.

always a typical scheme of the EEG recording: impedance checking, artifact elimination, cleaning the signal in the pre- and postprocessing phases, and exporting to the next steps of analysis.

3.9.3 GeoSource

Having the signal recorded, one can think about doing, for example, the source localization. The GeoSource[5] software was developed by EGI and is an option in the EGI laboratory system. It can solve the EEG inverse problem, and it calculates sources of the currents flowing through the medium, in this case through the subject's head. With the LORETA and sLORETA algorithms, one can generate the visualization of the activity propagation either in the head volume (including subcortical structures) or on the cortex of the so-called flat map with particular BA being highlighted during the activation.

Thus, it is possible to export to the data set the time of the occurrence of a given activation and the electric current in nanoamperes flowing throughout the

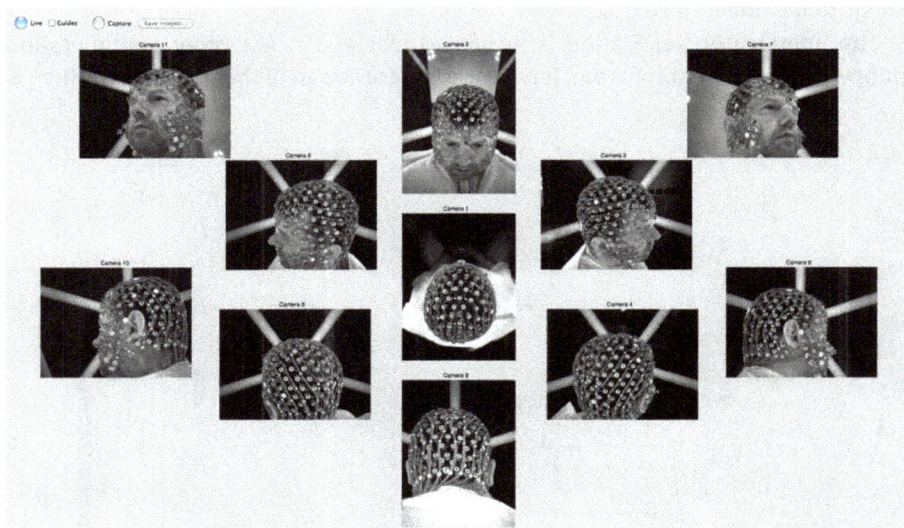

Fig. 3.5: Photos taken by 11 cameras of the photogrammetry station with Net Local software supporting GeoSource. When the subject leaves the laboratory, the assistant marks the black reference electrodes so that the GeoSource software could use the model of the subject's brain.

---

5 GeoSource 3 electrical source imaging packages: https://www.egi.com/research-division/electrical-source-imaging/geosource.

selected BA. To place the activity on the brain model with perfect accuracy, the lab should be equipped with a photogrammetry station. After selecting the referential electrodes in the photos taken by cameras placed in the photogrammetry gantry's corners, it is possible to generate the perfect model of the subject's head and, as mentioned above, to create a visualization of dipole propagation with the spatial resolution characteristic for the CT. Fig. 3.5 presents the photos taken by the photogrammetry station. The visualization mentioned above will be presented later in this chapter.

3.9.4 EEG lab

What happens if there is no access to the lab manufactured by EGI and accompanied by the Net Station and GeoSource software? It turns out that most of the cleaning, preprocessing, and postprocessing operations as well as the source localization can be conducted in the available free-of-charge and open source MATLAB toolbox. Similar to the closed and expensive solutions, the EEGLAB[6] [23] offers its own graphical user interface, multiformat data import, lots of plotting functions, semiautomated artifact removal, source modeling for both forward and inverse problems, ICA implementation, and the possibility to add external plug-ins. Visualizations generated in the EEGLAB toolbox are characteristic because of the rainbow-colored small head cross sections appearing in lots of papers in the last decades. The typical EEGLAB output is presented in Fig. 3.6.

3.9.5 Brainstorm

As far as the open source software is concerned, the best solution for neuroimaging and data visualization is offered by the Brainstorm[7] [24]. Not only the EEG signal can be totally processed by the Brainstorm but also other technologies, including MEG, MRI, and invasive experiment using animals. There is a very long list of amplifiers offered by practically all EEG equipment manufacturers that are supported by Brainstorm, and all leading brain atlases are compatible with 2D/3D models that can be generated in this environment. All the qEEG methods described in this chapter are supported, and most of the technical solutions used in the filtering or cleaning procedures are implemented at least as good as in the Net Station. It must be noted that using Brainstorm, it is possible to map the cortical electric activity recorded using EEG on the anatomical brain model generated by voxels obtained in MRI scan and including ultra-high-field frequency 7T scanners. Visualizations generated using

---

6 EEGLab: https://sccn.ucsd.edu/eeglab/.
7 Brainstorm: https://neuroimage.usc.edu/brainstorm/.

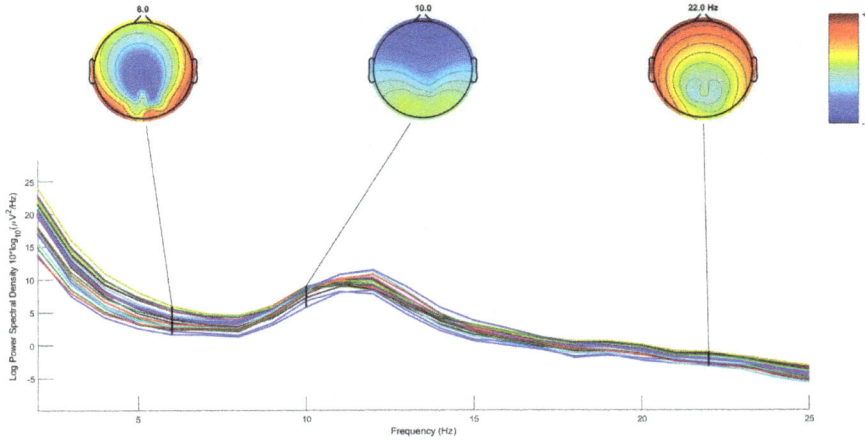

Fig. 3.6: Typical plots generated in the EEGLAB. Except for the rainbow cortical activity visualizations, one can observe the logarithm of power spectrum activity in the space of EEG in the frequency range from 0.1 to 25 Hz, generated using signal from the 26 most significant electrodes in some P300 experiment. (Courtesy of Andrzej Kawiak, MSc, Eng, CoNaBI)

Brainstorm are always very spectacular, and two examples are presented in Figs. 3.7 and 3.8.

3.10 Example of the Iowa Gambling Task experiment

Finally, we would like to present the example of the ERP experiment conducted in our laboratory, by showing its most important phases step by step. For example, we chose the Iowa Gambling Task (IGT).

Antoine Bechara, Antonio Damasio, Hanna Damasio, and Steven Anderson were the ones who brought the IGT into practice. Since that time, this activity has been one of the best liked by the subjects taking part in numerous experiments dealing with experimental psychology [25]. Based on the investigations, which were carried out for the first time at the Iowa University, the IGT was meant to control the decision-making process mechanisms applied in the card game with the reward-punishment orientation.

The rules of the game consist in choosing the deck symbol of one card out of four with 100 trials. The aim is to earn the most possible virtual money beginning with zero by the people taking part in it. Each set of four cards (or symbols) contains some good cards to be rewarded as well as some bad ones to be punished. However, not knowing which card is good and which one is bad, the participant must make a decision on the game course. The first impression is that all cards are good. However, the reward proves to be much higher when choosing two (of four) cards that seem to be better.

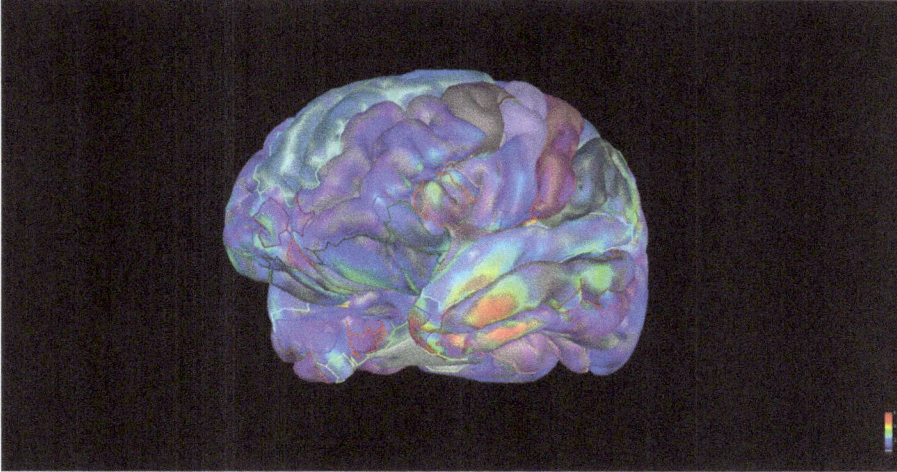

Fig. 3.7: Author's brain cortex visualization generated in Brainstorm. A 15-minute long meditation resting state is averaged and then presented. (Courtesy of Andrzej Kawiak, MSc, Eng, (CoNaBI))

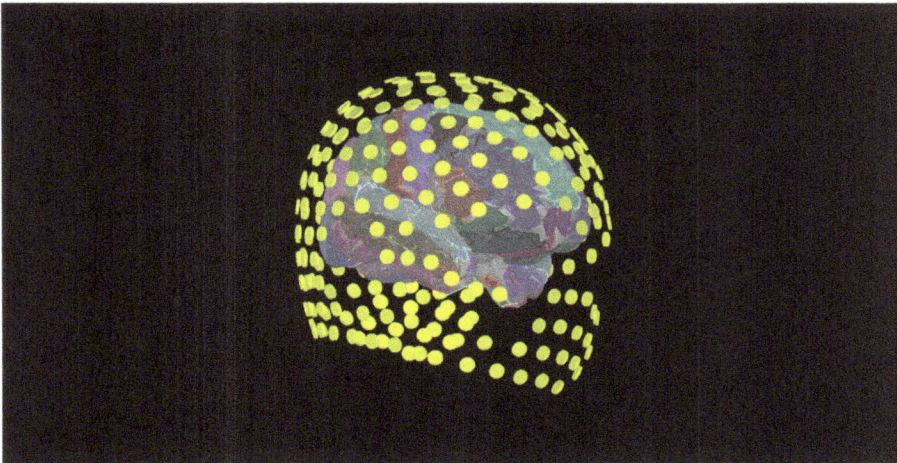

Fig. 3.8: Author's brain cortical activity with electrode position visualization generated in Brainstorm. During visualization, one can make any rotations of the model and check the activity of selected brain regions according to one of several most popular anatomical atlases of brain. (Courtesy of Andrzej Kawiak, MSc, Eng, (CoNaBI))

By choosing the better cards too many times, one is finally severely punished. However, the choice of the worse cards is mildly punished and, at the end of the game, results in better financial achievements in comparison with the other event. Fig. 3.9 shows the typical computer screen based on which decisions are made by participants.

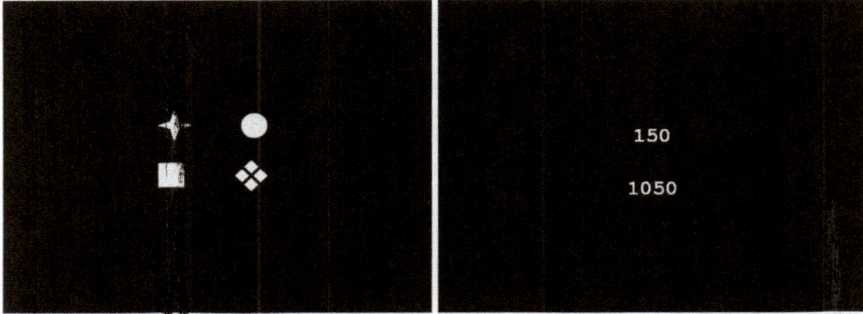

Fig. 3.9: Iowa Gambling Task typical screen shown to participant (in the left). He or she must choose one of four figures to receive awards and avoid punishments. Reward and total score are shown on the screen like that the right.

The case considered is when the subject signed the agreement to participate in the research and the EEG cap was placed on his head, which usually takes about 20 minutes. The cap consists of 256 electrodes, a moisture with an electrolyte that is kept in the bucket. Next, the impedance between the electrodes and the subject's scalp must be checked. The amplifier returns the information about the impedance, and if there are still some electrodes that do not contact the scalp properly, the electrolyte can be added to them without the necessity of taking the cap off. The abovementioned 100-trial series takes the subject about 15 minutes. Then the signal is recorded in the main laboratory computer system. After the signal recording, the subject is asked to get to the gantry of the photogrammetry station where the photos of his head in the EEG cap are taken (see Fig. 3.5). This is the last procedure applied to the subject in the lab. The preprocessing of the signal usually takes 2 hours. The laboratory worker must ensure that the signal is clean, without artifacts, and properly recorded. In the postprocessing phase, the additional several scripts must be applied to the signal. The names of the preprocessing and postprocessing scripts are similar in most software solutions and as follow the following: filtration, segmentation, artifact detection, manual signal cleaning, bad channel replacement, averaging, montage operations, and baseline correction. Each script, about which one can read in any software documentation, is responsible for the tasks that finally will enable the qEEG analysis. It should be remembered that to conduct good photogrammetry, the model of the brain must be generated by the Net Local software attached to the GPS system, and it is characteristic of that system, so there is no point in describing it in detail.

    The fragment of the raw EEG signal is presented in Fig. 3.10. One obtains 256 time series, each for one amplifier channel. Fig. 3.11 presents the power spectrum analysis for the selected channels. One can find the dominant frequencies in this selected time of the experiment. The DSM propagation appearing in the averaged signal is

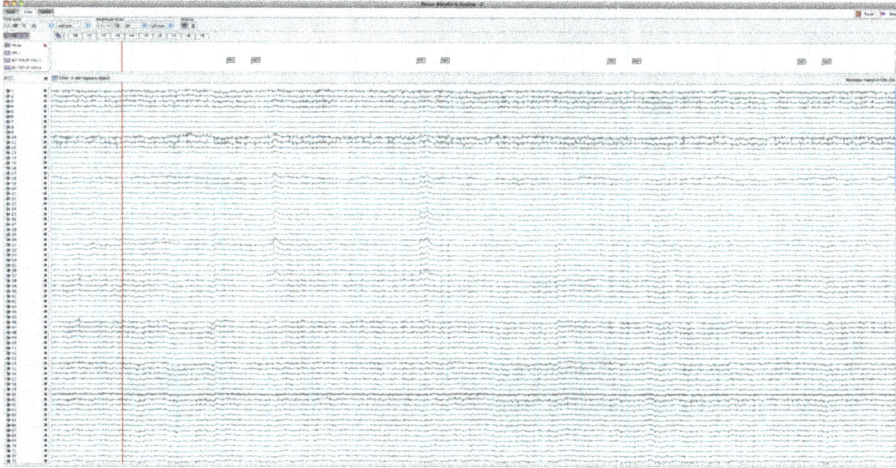

Fig. 3.10: Raw signal visible on the laboratory computer screen during the experiment. There is one plot for each of the 256 electrodes, varying in time. Although it is still far from drawing any conclusions on the basis of such a screen, it is possible to assess whether the signal is noisy or good.

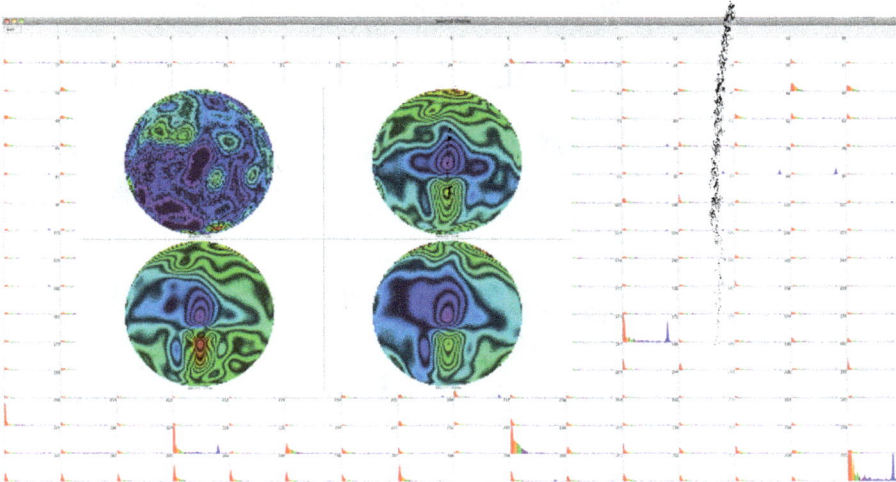

Fig. 3.11: During the experiment, it is possible to observe the Fourier analysis of the signal registered by particular electrodes. It is possible to save these data into separate data sets for further analysis.

presented in Fig. 3.12. The example of the frame from the sLORETA analysis conducted in the GeoSource is shown in subject's responses in Fig. 3.13.

It looks nice in the figures, but the raw signal takes several hundred gigabytes. To process one subject in the IGT, the researcher usually spends 12 hours. To arrange a

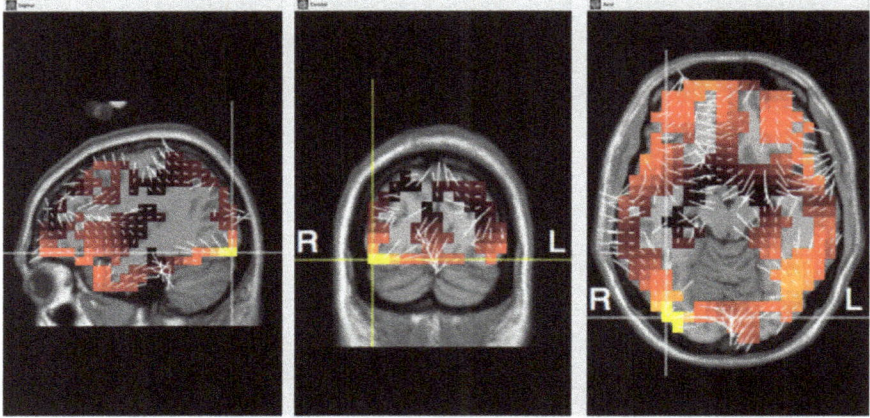

Fig. 3.12: Dipole propagation visualized in the GeoSource software in the discussed IGT experiment. The simulated activity is put on the brain model with CT-like resolution, and then it can be played as a movie.

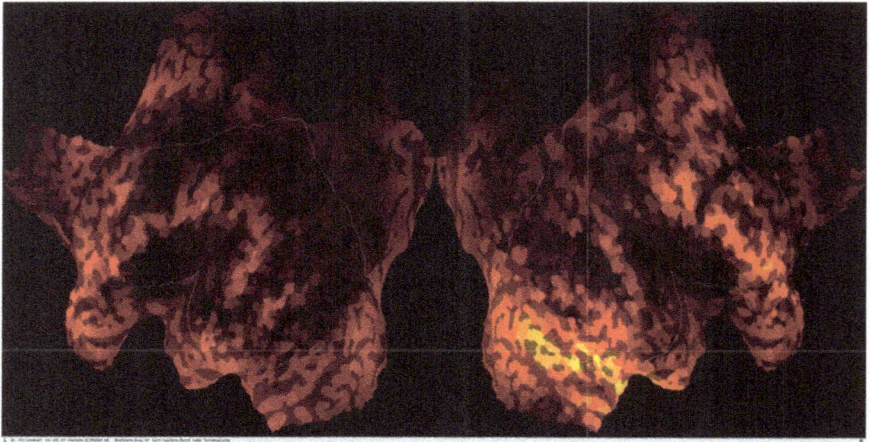

Fig. 3.13: Source localization calculated and later visualized using the GeoSource in the discussed IGT experiment. The simulated activity is presented in the so-called flat map of brain cortex with left (L in the left) and right (R in the right) hemispheres. Below one can read the activity of Brodmann area 11 and the intensity of 0.073880 nA, and Brodmann area 37 and the intensity of 0.290445 nA.

real experiment, we should consider at least 30 good recordings. Sometimes it is necessary to also build the control group. The EEG is an experimental science. In many cases, the signal of even 20% of participants cannot be processed properly. That is why we should consider larger cohorts than those mentioned above. Only having such a job done is it possible to prepare first scientific reports or papers.

3.11 Where do we go from here?

This chapter briefly describes, in our opinion, the most popular methods of quantitative analysis. One who has no experience in the EEG would ask the question, where should I go from here? There is no one clear answer. First of all, the readers who have access to the EEG laboratory and are eager to start doing the EEG ought to think of the experiment they intend to conduct. The decision whether to do the resting states or ERPs is fundamental. For sure, from both types, one gets hundreds of gigabytes of data. These data must be processed. All methods originating from the data science will be useful here. Thus, if the data science is involved in the EEG research, building appropriate hardware for the Big Data infrastructure should be taken into account. In the wide range of data science methods, the statistics and machine learning tools often play the key role. To support the researcher's workshop, it would be in demand to get some knowledge of the Python, Matlab, and R programming languages as well as some cloud architectures for the support. In each stage of research, the quality of the collected data and their security should be kept in mind as everything we record is very sensitive and legally protected. There are not many scientific areas in which so high interdisciplinary character, including IT, programming, data science, experimental psychology, and medicine, is manifested. Definitely, as the part of biomedical engineering area [26, 27], EEG and qEEG belong to that elite and interdisciplinary group [26, 27]. Probably that is why this is so fascinating.

3.12 References

[1] Finger S. *Origins of Neuroscience: A History of Explorations into Brain Function*. New York: Oxford University Press, 2001.
[2] Evans J. Abarbanel AM, eds. *Introduction to Quantitative EEG and Neurofeedback*. Elsevier, 1999.
[3] Caton R. "Electrical currents of the brain." *Journal of Nervous and Mental Disease* 2.4 (1875): 610.
[4] Berger H. "Über das elektrenkephalogramm des menschen." *European Archives of Psychiatry and Clinical Neuroscience* 87.1 (1929): 527–70.
[5] Beck A, Cybulski N. "Weitere untersuchungen über die elektrischen erscheinungen in der hirnrinde der affen und hunde." *Centralblatt für Physiologie* 1 (1892): 1–6.
[6] Beck A. "Die Bestimmung der localisation der gehirn-und ruckenmarksfunctionen vermittelst der elektrischen erscheinungen." *Centralblatt fur Physiologie* 4 (1890): 473–6.
[7] Kotyra S, Wojcik GM. "Steady state visually evoked potentials and their analysis with graphical and acoustic transformation." *Polish Conference on Biocybernetics and Biomedical Engineering*. Cham: Springer, 2017.
[8] Kotyra S, Wojcik GM. "The station for neurofeedback phenomenon research." *Polish Conference on Biocybernetics and Biomedical Engineering*. Cham: Springer, 2017.
[9] Wójcik GM, et al. "Usefulness of EGI EEG system in brain computer interface research." *Bio-Algorithms and Med-Systems* 9.2 (2013): 73–9.
[10] Kamarajan C, Porjesz B. "Advances in electrophysiological research." *Alcohol Research* 37, no. 1 (2015): 53.

[11] Luck SJ. *An Introduction to the Event-Related Potential Technique.* MIT Press, 2014.

[12] Wojcik GM, et al. "Mapping the human brain in frequency band analysis of brain cortex electroencephalographic activity for selected psychiatric disorders." *Frontiers in Neuroinformatics* 12 (2018).

[13] Wojcik GM, et al. "New protocol for quantitative analysis of brain cortex electroencephalographic activity in patients with psychiatric disorders." *Frontiers in Neuroinformatics* 12 (2018).

[14] Rose S, Ebersole JS. "Advances in spike localization with EEG dipole modeling." *Clinical EEG and Neuroscience* 40, no. 4 (2009): 281–7.

[15] Pascual-Marqui RD, et al. "Functional imaging with low-resolution brain electromagnetic tomography (LORETA): a review." *Methods and Findings in Experimental and Clinical Pharmacology* 24, Suppl C (2002): 91–5.

[16] Pascual-Marqui RD. "Standardized low-resolution brain electromagnetic tomography (sLORETA): technical details." *Methods and Findings in Experimental and Clinical Pharmacology* 24, Suppl D (2002): 5–12.

[17] Krishnaswamy P, et al. "Sparsity enables estimation of both subcortical and cortical activity from MEG and EEG." *Proceedings of the National Academy of Sciences* 114, no. 48 (2017): E10465–74.

[18] Jolliffe I. *Principal Component Analysis.* Springer Berlin Heidelberg, 2011.

[19] Hyvärinen A, Karhunen J, Oja E. *Independent Component Analysis.* Vol. 46. John Wiley & Sons, 2004.

[20] Gajos A, Wójcik GM. "Independent component analysis of EEG data for EGI system." *Bio-Algorithms and Med-Systems* 12, no. 2 (2016): 67–72.

[21] Gajos-Balińska A, Wójcik GM, Stpiczyński P. "High performance optimization of independent component analysis algorithm for EEG data." *International Conference on Parallel Processing and Applied Mathematics.* Cham: Springer, 2017.

[22] Gajos-Balinska A, Wojcik GM, Stpiczynski P. "Performance comparison of parallel fastICA algorithm in the PLGrid structures." *ITM Web of Conferences.* Vol. 21. EDP Sciences, 2018.

[23] Delorme A, Makeig S. "EEGLAB: an open source toolbox for analysis of single-trial EEG dynamics including independent component analysis." *Journal of Neuroscience Methods* 134, no. 1 (2004): 9–21.

[24] Tadel F, et al. "Brainstorm: a user-friendly application for MEG/EEG analysis." *Computational Intelligence and Neuroscience* 2011 (2011): 8.

[25] Bechara A, et al. "Insensitivity to future consequences following damage to human prefrontal cortex." *Cognition* 50, nos. 1–3 (1994): 7–15.

[26] Tadeusiewicz R, ed. *Neurocybernetyka Teoretyczna.* Wydawnictwa Uniwersytetu Warszawskiego, 2009.

[27] Tadeusiewicz R. "New trends in neurocybernetics." *Computer Methods in Materials Science* 10, no. 1 (2010): 1–7.

Anna Sochocka, Liwia Leś, and Rafał Starypan

4 The visualization of the construction of the human eye

4.1 Introduction

In the twenty-first century, the e-learning platforms and computer simulators of the human body revolutionized medicine science. Simulators, serious games, and virtual atlases contribute to the fact that studying medicine is no longer an arduous and boring duty but is becoming an incredible adventure, a virtual journey inside the human body that a young adept of medicine can repeat over and over without any concern about making a mistake that will result in an irreversible injury of a patient. Students of medicine prefer watching a three-dimensional medical exhibit on a computer screen rather than a flat photograph in a book. When a person does not have spatial imagination, such a virtual model is a very useful solution [1].

Contemporary facilities in medicine consist not only of professional computer models realized by modern graphics but mostly of animation, which, combined with graphics, provides an ideal tool that enables not only a student of medicine but also an ordinary patient to understand complicated medical issues. Nothing can develop imagination better than a moving image that reflects human organism in perfect detail. This enables patients without any medical preparation to understand processes taking place in their organisms.

Computer applications used in the process of studying medicine can bear the character of serious games as well as computer simulators that, using mathematical models saved as computer programs, emulate a self-played physical phenomenon. However, nowadays serious games are mostly video games whose main purpose is education through entertainment.

Clarc C. Abt phrased the idea of serious games in the book *Serious Games* in 1975. In the introduction, he claimed, "We develop serious games in such a way to give them a clear and well-thought educational aim and not to dedicate them mainly to entertainment."

This chapter is given over to an authorial educational game aimed to help in studying the anatomy and physiology of the human organ of sight and understanding the mechanics of vision. The game is supposed to support studying of the correct and pathological anatomy of the organ of sight. Its user can be a high school student as well as a medical student. The interaction in the game is organized in single player mode. Steering in the game is accessible using mouse and keyboard. The interface is based on the Polish language. Anatomical structures inside the game are described in Polish as well as in Latin. Specialist literature—textbooks [2–4] and anatomy atlas [5]—were used as a source of serious content. The basic, assumed method of studying is practicing skills. A player can take a test to check his/her new skills. Models made in 3ds Max program show the anatomy of the organ of sight in a very clear way, including, for example, the proportions of its particular structures or the positioning of these structures toward one another. The assumption was to enable a player to rotate the models intuitively, zoom, and divide into parts using a mouse to uncover the inner structures [1].

4.2 Overview of the existing solutions

The market offers many computer applications of the anatomic character enabling to study three-dimensional models of the human eye. These solutions can be payable as well as free. Some of them assume contractual anatomical precision. There are three samples of English-language anatomic applications presented in this chapter. They were chosen based on the quality of mapping of the anatomy and the functionality of the models. The first is the application created by Cyber Science 3D, which created its three-dimensional interactive version in cooperation with the publisher of one of the most popular anatomic atlases, *The Netter Atlas of Human Anatomy*. The atlas is available in a free beta version as well as in a paid version (14 days for free, then $5 monthly). None of them is dedicated to mobile devices. The free version allows to manipulate the model (rotating, zooming in/out, and unfolding into parts), check English names of particular elements, and make reference points visible. The application offers a lot of models depicting some parts of the human body [6].

The second of the presented applications is the application created by Anatronica Interactive Anatomy 3D, which can be used in an online version. (The browser must support the Unity Web Player plug-in. Also, a Flash technology version is available.) It can also be used after downloading a desktop Pro version (both of the versions are free of charge). The online version contains only a male model, whereas the Pro version contains a female model as well. Moreover, in the Pro version, models of better quality are used. In the application, all systems of the human body are available. On the model, the visibility and half-translucency of particular elements can be turned on/off, and the Latin names of those elements can be checked as well. The entire model can be rotated and zoomed in/out. In addition, there is a possibility of searching particular anatomical structures by their names, too. Finally, a user's knowledge can be checked by a test of single-choice questions. The last update of the project took place in December 2015 [7].

The last of the presented applications is the Eye—Practical Series by the 3D4Medical. Its aim is to help understand how the human eye works and what the vision defects and eye diseases consist in. The issues of the work of the eye and the concept of the refractive error are explained by 19 animations free of charge. Additional animations concern the eye diseases and the methods of treating them, but they are only available after the purchase from the level of the application. The cost of the application is $7.99. The animations can be stopped at an arbitrary moment, and a note/drawing with a pen can be made on the stopped picture. Moreover, there is an available interactive model of the eye, which can be used to check the names of particular structures (both English and Latin ones) as well as the pronunciation of these names. A user's knowledge can be tested using the quiz. It has two modes: the "drag and drop" and the test of multiple-choice questions [8].

4.3 Presentation of the written application

The design of the presented game assumed the execution of models of the correct and pathological anatomy of the organ of sight in full view as well as in cross section, enabling to see the sagittal plane [1]. The models of eyeball, muscles, nerves, and eye socket bones were performed using the 3ds Max program [9]. Their behaviors were programmed in Unity [10]. The development environment used while making the design was the MonoDevelop Unity. The pictures representing views seen by a patient with functional disorders of the organ of sight were edited using the Gimp program [11]. After starting the game, the user can choose one out of four options, which are marked with the following buttons: Model anatomiczny, Quiz, Przegląd zaburzeń, and Wyjście. Clicking the Model anatomiczny button takes the user to the part of the game where he/she can get familiarized with the correct anatomy of the eye. The presented model of the eye consists of the eye socket bone, muscles, nerves, eyeball, and other elements that cannot be counted to any of the above-mentioned categories. The user can display the model in full view (Fig. 4.1) or in hemisection showing the right part of the eye socket (Fig. 4.2). Switching between views is possible, thanks to the

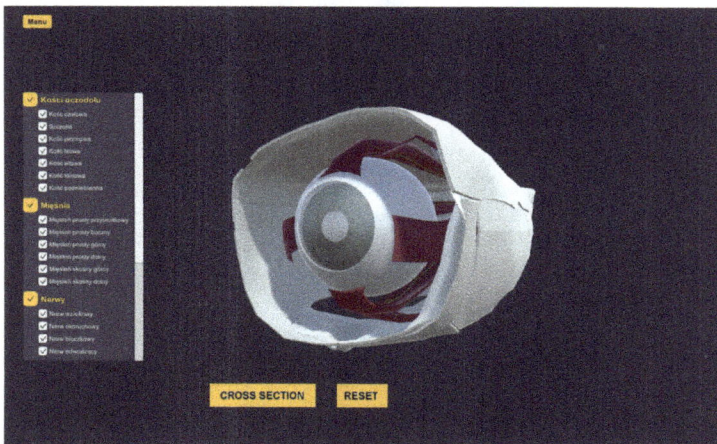

Fig. 4.1: The anatomic model window—full view [1].

buttons at the bottom of the screen. The model can be rotated using the arrow keys or W, S, A, and D keys as well as zoomed in/out with a scroll of a computer mouse.

Pointing a particular element with a mouse pointer makes it highlighted in blue and displays its name at the top of the screen (Fig. 4.2).

Pressing the space key while a particular structure is highlighted allows to separate it and deactivate other elements of the model. Moreover, at the same time, the description of this structure is displayed on the right side of the screen (Fig. 4.3). Clicking the right mouse button allows to go back to the previous window [1].

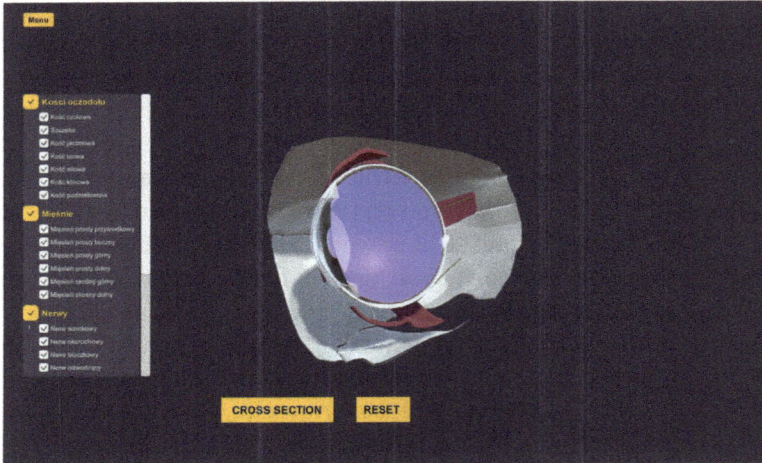

Fig. 4.2: The anatomic model window—hemisection [1].

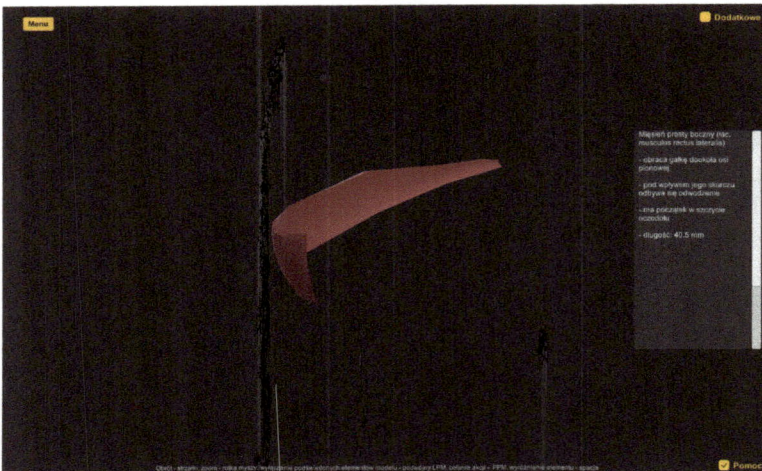

Fig. 4.3: The anatomic model window—distinction of a structure [1].

The game allows to view the inner structures of the organ of sight, too. The player can do it in two ways—by double clicking the left mouse button or by selecting an appropriate switch in the menu panel on the left side of the screen. The action can be withdrawn by clicking the right mouse button or by selecting an appropriate switch in the menu panel. Clicking any of the following buttons *Kości oczodołu (Eye socket bones)*, *Mięśnie (Muscles)*, *Nerwy (Nerves)*, *Gałka oczna (Eyeball)*, and *Inne (Other)* causes accordingly turn-on or turn-off of all of the elements of the model that belong to the particular category (Fig. 4.4) [1].

The main button marked as *Quiz* takes the user to the quiz window. At the beginning, the user is asked to choose the language in which the names of the anatomical structures during the quiz will be presented. There are two options to choose from—Polish or Latin (Fig. 4.5a). At the end of the quiz, the user is informed about the result that he/she obtained (Fig. 4.5b, c). The test can be repeated or a new test can be taken [1].

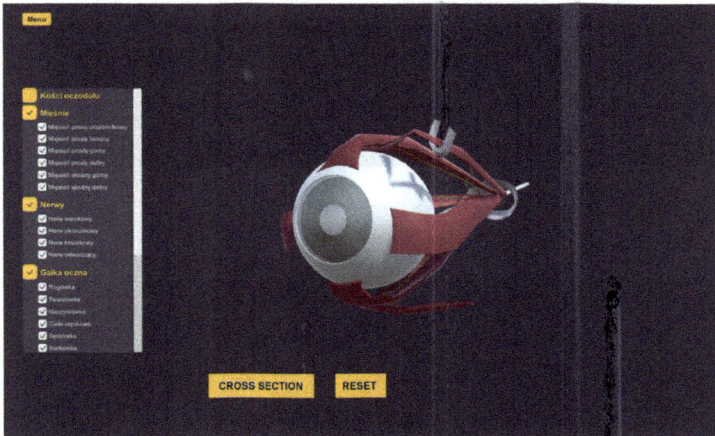

Fig. 4.4: The anatomic model window—the eye socket bones tuned off [1].

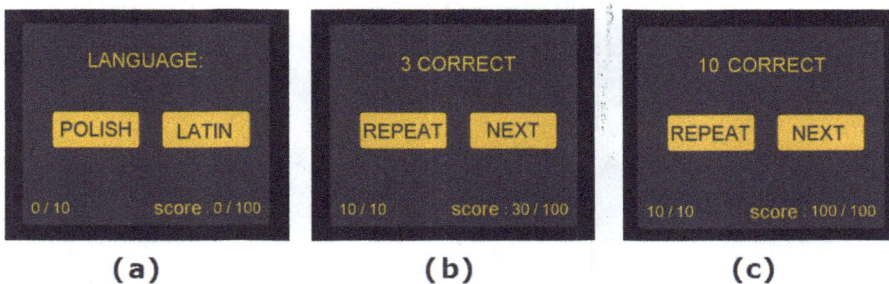

Fig. 4.5: Extracts of the quiz window: (a) choice of the language, (b and c) the end of the quiz [1].

Each quiz consists of 10 questions in which one out of four answers should be marked. While solving the quiz, the number of the question and the result obtained so far are displayed under the current question (Figs. 4.6 and 4.7) [1].

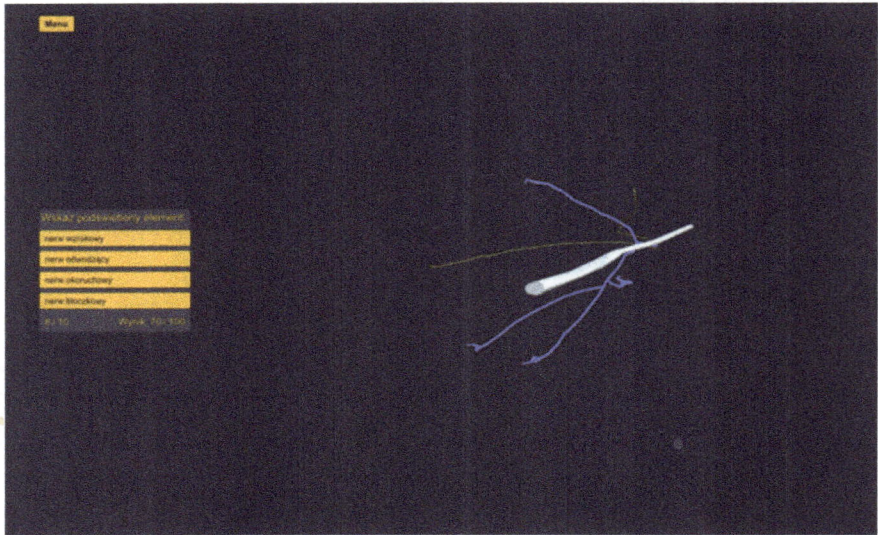

Fig. 4.6: The quiz window—questions concerning Polish terminology [1].

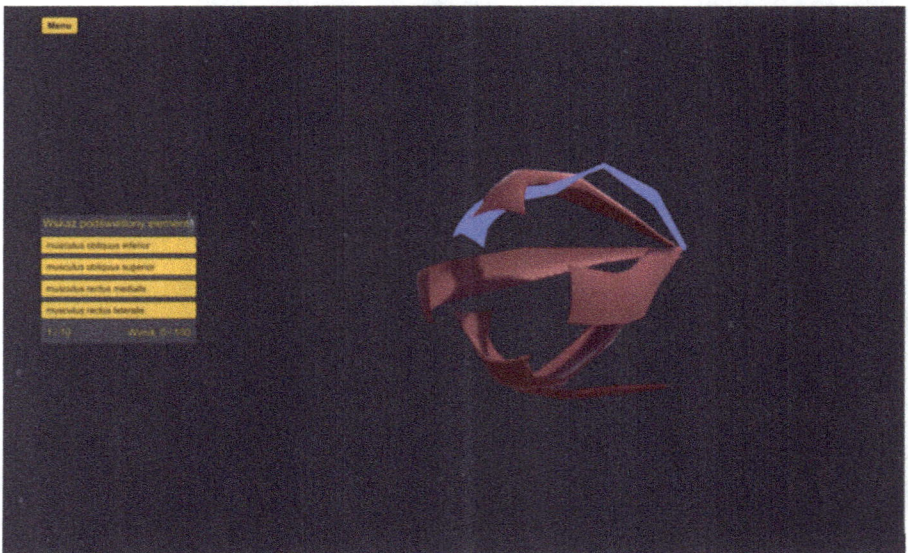

Fig. 4.7: The quiz window—questions concerning Latin terminology [1].

The last option available is the *Przegląd zaburzeń (Overview of disorders)* button that takes the user to the part of the game dedicated to disorders of the organ of sight. The user can get familiarized with three eyesight defects and four diseases [1]. The application allows to get familiarized with particular defects and the way of perceiving the world by a person with such a defect. Figs. 4.8 and 4.9 present the disorder panel of myopia and astigmatism.

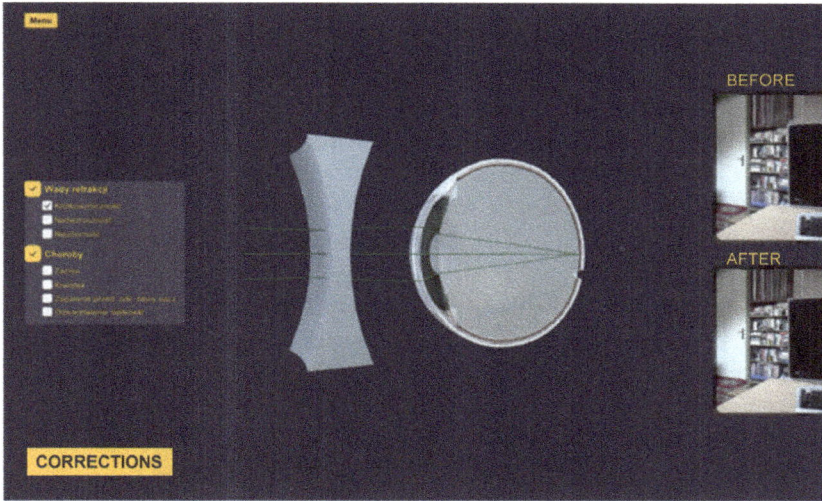

Fig. 4.8: The window for disorder of myopia "before" and "after" correction [1].

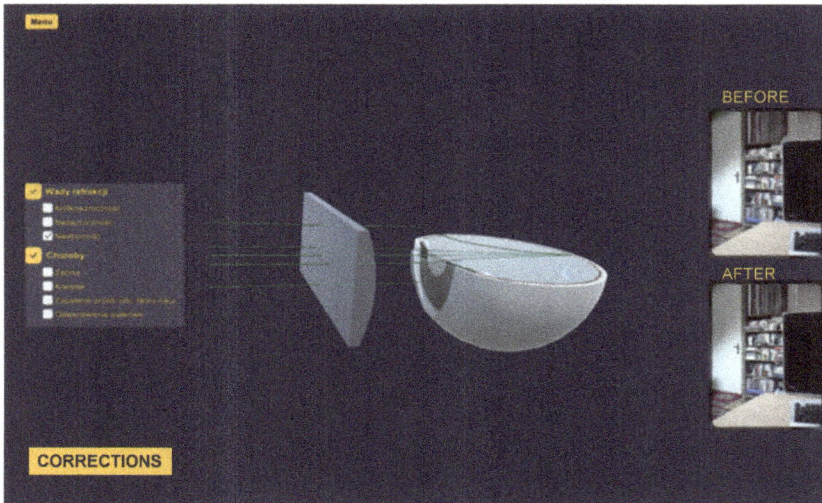

Fig. 4.9: The window for disorder of astigmatism "before" and "after" correction [1].

The user can always go back to the main menu after clicking the "Menu" button, which is visible in the upper left corner of the screen or pressing the "Esc" key. The application can be quit after clicking the "Wyjście" (Quit) button.

4.4 Summary

The presented game belongs to the category of serious games in which the main role is to teach through playing. The demonstrated application is dedicated to pupils, students, and all other persons who are interested in getting acquainted with anatomy of the human eye and defects of the organ of sight. In the future, the game can be extended by elements of a model of the correct anatomy (of e.g., lacrimal apparatus, conjunctivas, eyelids, and vascularity) as well as by a greater number of defects and diseases. The application was tested by second-year medical students at the Jagiellonian University Medical College within the course "Simulation in Medicine." The students did not report any negative remarks, their attitude was rather positive, and they expressed an interest in the subject. They were of the opinion that it was an interesting alternative to medical picture dictionaries, and learning through playing is an interesting solution.

Based on these remarks, it can be concluded that serious games are the future of science and, for certain, an interesting alterative to classic handbooks.

4.5 References

[1] Leś L. "Wizualizacja pracy ludzkiego oka." Mater's thesis at WFAIS UJ.

[2] Lens A, CoyneNemeth S, Ledford JK. *Anatomia i fizjologia narządu wzroku*. Wrocław: Górnicki Wydawnictwo Medyczne, 2010.

[3] Herba E, Pojda SM, Pojda-Wilczek D, Zatorska B. *Okulistyka w kropelce*. Katowice: Śląska Akademia Medyczna, 2006.

[4] Niżankowska MH. *Okulistyka. Podstawy kliniczne*. Warszawa: Wydawnictwo Lekarskie PZWL, 2007.

[5] Paulsen F, Waschke J. *Sobotta Atlas of Human Anatomy, Head, Neck and Neuroanatomy*. München: Urban & Fischer, 2011.

[6] *Information on the 'Netter 3D Anatomy'*. http://netter3danatomy.com/ (last access October 10, 2019).

[7] Information on the products of the *'Anatronica Interactive Anatomy 3D'* company. http://www.anatronica.com/ (last access August 10, 2017).

[8] Information on the *'Eye – Practical Series'*. http://3d4medical.com/apps/eye-practical-series (last access 10.08.17r.).

[9] *Information on the 3ds Max program*. http://www.tutorialboneyard.com/3ds-max-introduction/ (last access October 10, 2019).

[10] Smith M, Queiroz C. *Unity 5.x Cookbook*. Birmingham: Packt Publishing, 2015.

[11] *Information on the Gimp program*. https://www.gimp.org/ (last access October 10, 2019).

Jan Witowski, Mateusz Sitkowski, Mateusz K. Hołda,
and Michał Pędziwiatr

5 Three-dimensional printing in preoperative and intraoperative decision making

5.1 Introduction

The expansion of minimally invasive surgery and transcatheter interventions put greater meaning on imaging techniques in patient qualification and procedure planning. For better understanding of the anatomy on standard volumetric medical images, modern three-dimensional (3D) visualization methods have found to be especially beneficial. They include 3D printing, augmented and virtual reality, or advanced rendering techniques, such as cinematic rendering. The major advantages of 3D printing above other methods include element of tactility, which makes the experience more realistic for the surgeon, and ability to simulate procedures. Having said that, there is no strong evidence right now whether there are differences between those techniques in terms of clinical outcomes or decision making.

This chapter will introduce basic concepts of 3D printing, overview of methodology, and state of the art in current clinical practice. We will put special attention to real-life cases where 3D printing is being implemented routinely for preoperative and intraoperative decision making. This chapter covers only the main field of clinical 3D printing, which consists of personalized anatomical models. We will not discuss topics related to 3D printed implants, dental 3D printing, or bioprinting.

5.2 Introduction of 3D printing to clinical practice

Although 3D printing has its history reaching back to 1980s and first attempts to use it in medicine were in the 1990s and early 2000s (especially in the U.S. military), truly clinical 3D printing started in 2008 in Mayo Clinic in Rochester, MN, USA. This case and establishing the first clinical 3D printing lab at Mayo's Department of Radiology by Jonathan Morris and Jane Matsumoto in 2013 were the starting points to the great expansion of clinical 3D printing [1]. Initial reports and reviews suggested extremely high benefits of using the technology and broad range of possible implementations in all medical fields [2, 3]. However, just within next few years, researchers have found areas that can gain from 3D printing the most and quickly experimented with it. So far, orthopedics, maxillofacial surgery, and cardiology have been the fields with most 3D printed models. Anatomical models and surgical guides are the most common types of printouts. These initial reports, though, have helped to move the field forward quickly. Special interest groups and working teams within societies were created, with

Radiological Society of North America (RSNA) in the front. Currently, it unites several hundred medical professionals and researchers working on 3D printing.

It is important to notice that although 3D printing is available for about a decade now, clinical evidence is still relatively sparse. The most published research consists of case studies, as the personalization of 3D printing comes most useful in rare and complex cases. The first meta-analyses have been published very recently, virtually only in orthopedic surgery [4, 5]. Systematic reviews have been performed for most medical fields, however, and have shown that models are accurate and helpful. Having said that, those conclusions are drawn usually just from physicians' reports and with no quantitative data to support it. In-hospital 3D printing labs are still located in almost only large university hospitals, often with industry support. There is a slow change toward more desktop, user-friendly, and accessible machines, and the process itself is simplifying, helping the expansion of the technology. It is still most likely that smaller, rural hospitals will never need 3D printing services.

5.3 The 3D printing process

There are many definitions for 3D printing. To simplify, it can be described as fabricating physical 3D object based on virtual 3D mesh, by successively printing layers on top of one another. In medical scenario, "physical 3D object" is usually an anatomical model, and "virtual 3D mesh" is a computer representation of anatomical structure. The crucial part of clinical 3D printing, however, is the process that leads to creating that virtual model based on medical imaging. This process, called *segmentation*, has been widely explored in computer vision for decades, which led to partial automatization [6]. Several open-source software packages are available to speed up segmentation process with access to semiautomatic algorithms, e.g., thresholding or region growing. Having said that, segmentation is still considered one of the main bottlenecks of 3D visualization and 3D printing processes.

The idea of segmentation is simple: anatomical regions of interests (ROIs) have to be annotated (contoured) slice by slice, preferably by an expert in medical imaging. Today, it is a common practice in medical 3D printing labs to have a team of engineers performing segmentations and have them reviewed and confirmed by experienced radiologists. This task, depending on body area and quality of imaging, can take anywhere from 1 min to 5 h. Good examples of more complex cases are as follows: visceral anatomy (hepatic veins, renal vasculature), tumors with heterogenous attenuation, and vague borders, nerves, or lymph nodes. Segmented ROIs can be exported as "masks" or "labelmaps," usually in binary format (0, background; 1, area of interest), relative pixelwise to input data. They can also be easily exported straight to virtual 3D mesh, usually in .stl or .obj formats, and subsequently displayed—this process is called *surface rendering*. Once the mesh is exported, it—theoretically—is ready to be 3D printed. However, some sort of postprocessing is usually performed before sending files to a printer. The most common postprocessing operations are making the model hollow, cutting through the model, dividing model into several parts, smoothing, and adding identifiers or text onto the mesh. There is a final step before the model can be 3D printed. Files with models have to be loaded into the software that is handling communication with the printer and "translating the mesh language into 3D printer language." The language of 3D printers (and other CNC machines), called *G-code*, consists of instructions on how to create physical 3D object layer by layer. This translation from 3D mesh to G-code is sometimes referred to as *slicing*, and software packages are called *slicers*. Although for most 3D printers there are dedicated, proprietary solutions, some open-source slicers are available. The most commonly used currently are Cura (open-source) and Simplify3D (Fig. 5.1). (Note: do not confuse *slicers* with 3D Slicer—popular open-source software for segmentation that does not perform *slicing* for 3D printing.)

Again, physical 3D objects are created by successively printing layers on top of one another. There are a number of methods that make it possible; however, they usually are based on two ideas: melting hard filaments or solidification of liquid or powder. The first method uses filaments (usually polylactic acid [PLA] or acrylonitrile

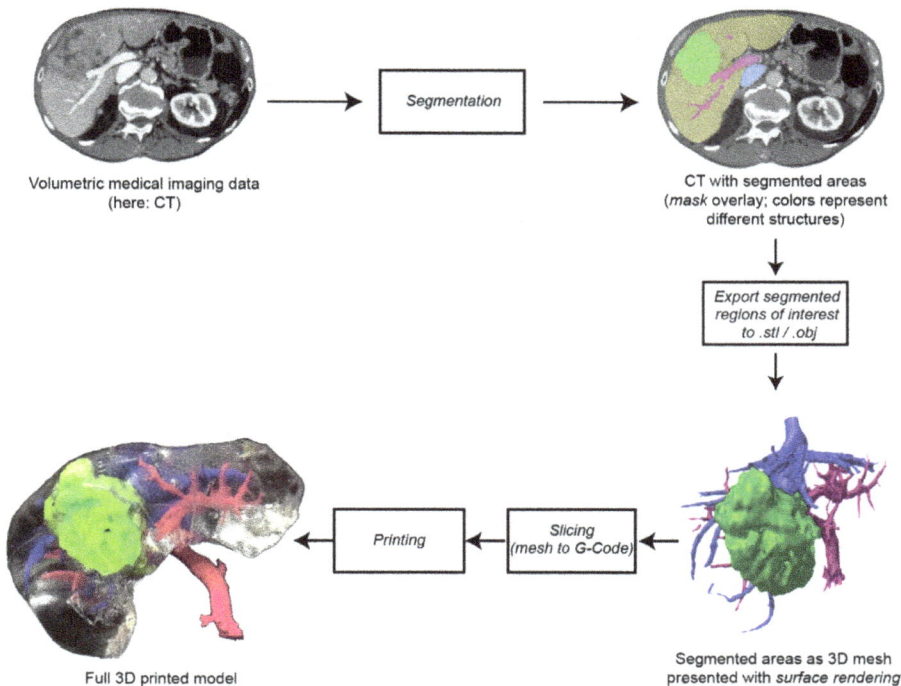

Fig. 5.1: Workflow of 3D printing: all phases from image acquisition to printed model. Case of 3D printing liver models for preoperative planning, done routinely at Jagiellonian University (Kraków, Poland).

butadiene styrene [ABS]) that are being heated up in printer and disposed layer by layer through a nozzle. Filament solidifies just after extrusion as it cools off, forming a 3D structure. The second approach uses fluids (usually resins) solidified with UV light or powder solidified with laser beam. Is it important to know the trade-off between all methods. Some of them may not be useful in specific clinical applications (Fig. 5.2, Tab. 5.1).

5.4 Clinical example: liver models

Laparoscopic liver surgery is often the treatment of choice for patients with intra-hepatic malignancies. Those procedures require extensive preoperative workup,

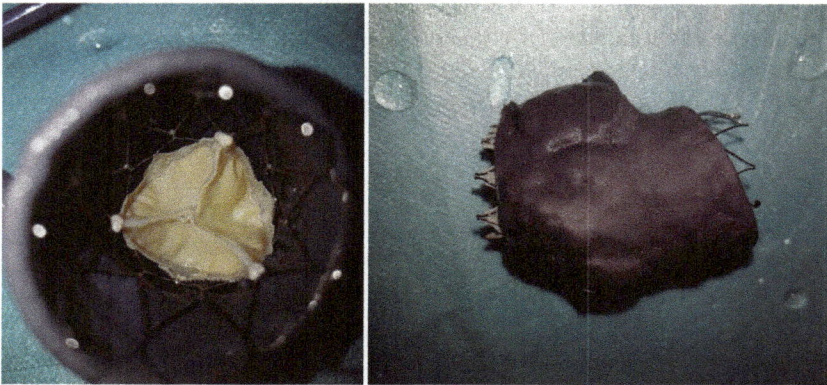

Fig. 5.2: Model of aortic root 3D printed with stereolithography technique. Semiflexible resin allowed the simulation of transcatheter aortic valve implantation (TAVI) and proper valve sizing. Model was created in 2017 for cardiologists from Warsaw Medical University (Warsaw, Poland).

Tab. 5.1: Comparison of the most common 3D printing fabrication methods

	Fused deposition modeling (FDM)	**Stereolithography (SLA; or DLP)**	**Selective later sintering (SLS)**	**"PolyJet"/"multicolor printing"**
Printing method	Melting hard filaments	Solidifying fluid	Solidifying powder	Solidifying fluid
Costs	Very low	Low/medium	Medium/high	Extremely high
Materials	Very limited, virtually no flexible materials	From tough to slightly flexible	From tough to very flexible	From tough to very flexible
Clinical potential	Good visualization potential, low simulation potential	Good visualization potential, medium simulation potential	Medium visualization potential, good simulation potential	Very good visualization and simulation potential

including imaging (computed tomography or magnetic resonance) and precise planning. Understanding 3D relationships between tumors and hepatic vessels is crucial in performing safe and effective resections. As laparoscopic hepatectomies are elective procedures, 3D printing seems perfect as an aid in decision making.

There are approximately 20 studies published in the area of liver surgery [7, 8]. Most of them, unfortunately, are case studies or case series. As liver models require visualization of multiple structures at once, PolyJet is the fabrication method of choice in most cases, although cost-effective approaches are also explored [9]. Our research group has also shown that 3D printed liver models are highly accurate [10]. A 2019 study by Yang et al. [11] presents that printed models result in the improved assessment of tumor location in comparison with MDCT and standard virtual 3D reconstruction. They also proved that understanding 3D relationship is easier with printed model, as time spent on assessing the tumor location was lowest between all groups (93 s in 3D printing group, over 200 s in other two). Unfortunately, no large randomized or standard prospective trials have been published yet. Our group is running a clinical trial (registered in ClinicalTrials.gov database under NCT03744624 identifier), which is aimed to recruit approximately 85 patients and end before the end of 2022.

Three-dimensional printing in liver surgery is a great example of difficulties related to getting strong evidence of clinical benefits. Patient group is very heterogenic, and getting statistically significant results requires the recruitment of a large number of individuals. Liver models are also more costly and require more work than others because they have to be multimaterial and multicolor for full immersion. PolyJet-based liver models can cost up to a few thousand dollars per one model [12]. Low-cost methods can reduce this to approximately $150, although they require more manpower and time. In oncological patients qualified for resection, these models are extremely helpful in choosing the most optimal resection plane and establishing safe resection margins. Preoperative decision making can reduce number of alterations to surgical plan during complex procedure and may help in finding patients who are most exposed to posthepatectomy liver failure. Trial results in coming years should answer whether this is the case (Fig. 5.3).

5.5 Clinical example: congenital heart disease and transcatheter interventions

Congenital heart disease printed models are one of the most explored and proven applications of medical 3D printing. There are a number of studies proving its utility and several labs dedicated to work specifically in this area (Fig. 5.4).

In 2018, the RSNA 3D Printing Special Interest Group published their first guidelines on clinical use of 3D printing. Guidelines included congenital heart disease, craniomaxillofacial, genitourinary, musculoskeletal, vascular, and breast 3D

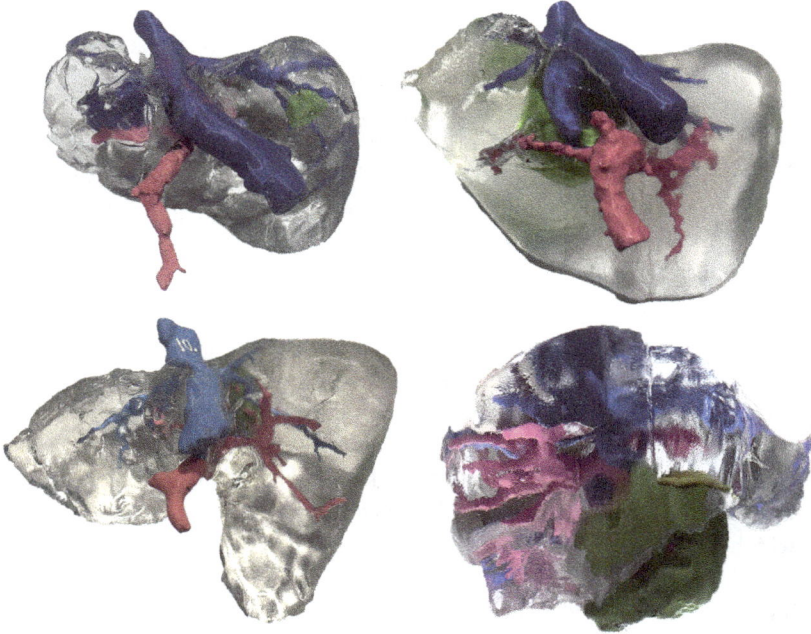

Fig. 5.3: Examples of 3D liver models, developed routinely at Jagiellonian University (Kraków, Poland). They are fully personalized, full sized, and multimaterial. Our unique low-cost approach allowed to reduce production from approximately $2,000 to $150 per model. Average time from CT acquisition to model delivery is 5 days. Transparent parenchyma is made with silicone by casting it into a mold printed on a desktop FDM 3D printer.

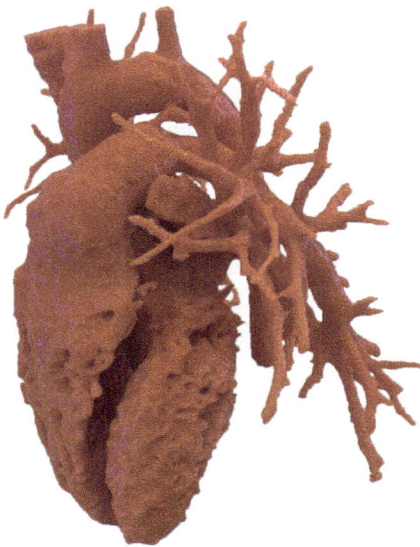

Fig. 5.4: Fused deposition modeling approach allows labs to create personalized models of congenital heart diseases with approximately 24-h turnaround time from image acquisition. This fabrication technique was satisfactory here, as models are used only for visualization and not for simulation. The model in this picture was delivered to cardiologists from University Children's Hospital of Kraków.

models [13]. Appropriateness Guidelines scored medical conditions on a scale from 1 to 10 (10 being most useful and with strongest clinical evidence). Double outlet right ventricle, truncus arteriosus, and anomalous pulmonary venous connection were the conditions found to benefit the most from 3D printing and scored 8 and above. Surprisingly, arterial and ventricular septal defects scored very low, between 2 and 5, although 3D printed models have been proven to be very useful in simulating closure procedures. Flexible models of septal defects can be used to perform mock transcatheter procedures and may help in choosing proper device size, improving the safety of surgery [14]. They help to understand spatial relationships between structures normally seen by cardiologists in echocardiography and learn how to proceed with the catheter delivery system. Models for nonvalvular structural heart diseases, usually meaning left atrial appendage occlusion, help in choosing the proper device, similarly to septal defects.

At Jagiellonian University, we have created an "atlas" of 3D printed congenital heart disease models. Based on real cases and imaging, they show variability within a single condition. The atlas can be used for parent and patient education and for getting an informed consent. More complex models may also be available for less experienced cardiology and cardiac surgery residents for learning complex repair procedures. Although structures are relatively small, the resolution of 3D printers is high enough to make accurate representations of the anatomy. In addition, models can be scaled and divided in any way, providing many possibilities for visualization at request. Segmentation can be tricky, as mentioned before, although there is commercial software dedicated for cardiovascular segmentation, e.g., Mimics (Materialise NV, Leuven, Belgium), that can make this part as quick as 30 min. Elastic or multimaterial and multicolor models are preferred, although in our experience even rigid and monocolor models are useful.

Research shows that 3D printed cardiovascular models can be as effective in educational setting as cadaveric specimens, offering a way to avoid ethical issues. In some cases, they have also been proven to have similar mechanical properties and echocardiography visualization [15].

5.6 Creating in-house 3D lab and summary

There are multiple challenges necessary to consider when planning a new 3D printing in-hospital lab. Considering the budget, it is often forgotten that 3D printing is a work-consuming process, and it requires engagement of qualified people. Clinicians, preferably radiologists, should perform or at least review segmentations before model printing. Engineers should be able to properly choose the fabrication method to meet physician expectations and have a good insight into hardware. Three-dimensional printing is still fairly experimental, so it is safe to assume that some percentage of prints will either fail or not meet clinical expectations. The location of the lab is important too. To maintain maximum safety by avoiding fumes and fire risk, the lab should be well ventilated and separate from the clinical area. It is crucial to ask surgeons for intraoperative photo.

In medical 3D printing field, it is now clear that this technology will benefit both patients and clinicians. However, it will not be used everywhere and will not dramatically change the landscape. It seems that in the future, we will see more focus on simulations and preprocedural planning with 3D printing and routine use of it in complex cases. Advances in segmentation software and further reduction of costs related to 3D printers should automatize the process and make it more accessible to smaller institutions, especially outside the United States (Fig. 5.5).

We have not discussed topics related to ethical and legal issues. For example, who is the owner of a patient's data? Do we consider 3D models or printers equipment requiring FDA approval? For more information on this, please refer to FDA's Technical

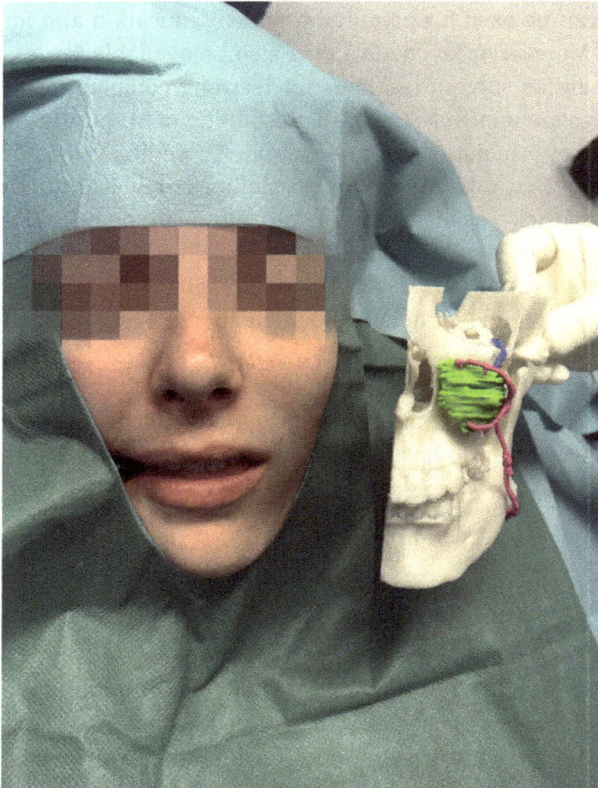

Fig. 5.5: Intraoperative photo of 3D printed facial lesion model with close proximity to facial artery and infraorbital nerve. Created with fused deposition modeling approach, was used by plastic surgeons in Wrocław, Poland.

Considerations for Additive Manufactured Medical Devices, which is currently the only official guideline from U.S. government bodies regarding medical 3D printing [16] as well as James Coburn and Gerald Grant [17] commentary on the FDA process. We have also omitted validation and verification issues: there is no standardization is this area. The largest 3D printing labs have established their own, internal quality assessment protocols. Please refer to a chapter written by Dimitrios Mitsouras, Elizabeth George, and Frank Rybicki [18] to learn more about this. There are also strong efforts in several 3D printing working groups, especially RSNA 3DP SIG, toward assuring high model accuracy and quality.

5.7 References

[1] Matsumoto, Jane S, Jonathan M. Morris, Thomas A. Foley, Eric E. Williamson, Shuai Leng, Kiaran P. McGee, Joel L. Kuhlmann, Linda E. Nesberg, Terri J. Vrtiska. "Three-dimensional physical modeling: applications and experience at Mayo Clinic." *Radiographics* 35, no. 7 (2015): 1989–2006.

[2] Ventola, Lee C. "Medical applications for 3D printing: current and projected uses." *Pharmacy and Therapeutics* 39, no. 10 (2014): 704–11. http://www.ncbi.nlm.nih.gov/pmc/articles/PMC4189697/.

[3] Rengier F, Mehndiratta A, Von Tengg-Kobligk H, Zechmann CM, Unterhinninghofen R, Kauczor HU, Giesel FL. "3D printing based on imaging data: review of medical applications." *International Journal of Computer Assisted Radiology and Surgery* 5, no. 4 (2010): 335–41. https://doi.org/10.1007/s11548-010-0476-x.

[4] Zhang YD, Wu RY, Xie DD, Zhang L, He Y, Zhang H. "Effect of 3D printing technology on pelvic fractures: a meta-analysis." *Zhongguo Gu Shang = China Journal of Orthopaedics and Traumatology* 31, no. 5 (2018): 465–71.

[5] Bai, Jianzhong, Yongxiang Wang, Pei Zhang, Meiying Liu, Peian Wang, Jingcheng Wang, Yuan Liang. "Efficacy and safety of 3D print-assisted surgery for the treatment of pilon fractures: a meta-analysis of randomized controlled trials." *Journal of Orthopaedic Surgery and Research* 13, no. 1 (2018): 283. https://doi.org/10.1186/s13018-018-0976-x.

[6] Pal, Nikhil R, Sankar K. Pal. "A review on image segmentation techniques." *Pattern Recognition* 26, no. 9 (1993): 1277–94. https://doi.org/https://doi.org/10.1016/0031-3203(93)90135-J.

[7] Witowski, Jan Sylwester, Jasmine Coles-Black, Tomasz Zbigniew Zuzak, Michal Pędziwiatr, Jason Chuen, Piotr Major, Andrzej Budzyński. "3D printing in liver surgery: a systematic review." *Telemedicine Journal and E-Health : The Official Journal of the American Telemedicine Association* 23, no. 12 (2017): 943–47. https://doi.org/10.1089/tmj.2017.0049.

[8] Perica, Elizabeth Rose, Zhonghua Sun. "A systematic review of three-dimensional printing in liver disease." *Journal of Digital Imaging* 31, no. 5 (2018): 692–701. https://doi.org/10.1007/s10278-018-0067-x.

[9] Witowski, Jan Sylwester, Michał Pędziwiatr, Piotr Major, Andrzej Budzyński. "Cost-effective, personalized, 3D-printed liver model for preoperative planning before laparoscopic liver hemihepatectomy for colorectal cancer metastases." *International Journal of Computer Assisted Radiology and Surgery* 12, no. 12 (2017): 2047–54. https://doi.org/10.1007/s11548-017-1527-3.

[10] Witowski, Jan, Nicole Wake, Anna Grochowska, Zhonghua Sun, Andrzej Budzynski, Piotr Major, Tadeusz Jan Popiela, Michal Pedziwiatr. "Investigating accuracy of 3d printed liver models with computed tomography." *Quantitative Imaging in Medicine and Surgery 9*, no. 1 (2019): 43–52. https://doi.org/10.21037/qims.2018.09.16.

[11] Yang, Tianyou, Shuwen Lin, Qigen Xie, Wenwei Ouyang, Tianbao Tan, Jiahao Li, Zhiyuan Chen, et al. "Impact of 3D printing technology on the comprehension of surgical liver anatomy." *Surgical Endoscopy 33*, no. 2 (2019): 411–17. https://doi.org/10.1007/s00464-018-6308-8.

[12] Zein, Nizar N, Ibrahim A. Hanouneh, Paul D. Bishop, Maggie Samaan, Bijan Eghtesad, Cristiano Quintini, Charles Miller, Lisa Yerian, Ryan Klatte. "Three-dimensional print of a liver for preoperative planning in living donor liver transplantation." *Liver Transplantation 19* (2013): 1304–10. https://doi.org/10.1002/lt.23729.

[13] Chepelev, Leonid, Nicole Wake, Justin Ryan, Waleed Althobaity, Ashish Gupta, Elsa Arribas, Lumarie Santiago, et al. "Radiological Society of North America (RSNA) 3D Printing Special Interest Group (SIG): guidelines for medical 3D printing and appropriateness for clinical scenarios." *3D Printing in Medicine 4*, no. 1 (2018): 11. https://doi.org/10.1186/s41205-018-0030-y.

[14] Yan, Chaowu, Cheng Wang, Xiangbin Pan, Shiguo Li, Huijun Song, Qiong Liu, Nan Xu, Jianpeng Wang. "Three-dimensional printing assisted transcatheter closure of atrial septal defect with deficient posterior–inferior rim." *Catheterization and Cardiovascular Interventions 92*, no. 7 (2018): 1309–14. https://doi.org/10.1002/ccd.27799.

[15] Sabbagh, Abdallah El, Mackram F. Eleid, Mohammed Al-hijji, Nandan S. Anavekar, David R. Holmes, Vuyisile T. Nkomo, Gustavo S. Oderich, et al. "The various applications of 3D printing in cardiovascular diseases," *Current Cardiology Reports 20* (2018): 1–9. https://doi.org/10.1007/s11886-018-0992-9.

[16] U.S. Food and Drug Administration. *Technical Considerations for Additive Manufactured Medical Devices. Guidance for Industry and Food and Drug Administration Staff.* Silver Spring, MD: Center for Biologics Evaluation and Research, 2017. https://www.fda.gov/media/97633/download.

[17] Coburn, James C, Gerald T. Grant. "FDA regulatory pathways and technical considerations for the 3D printing of medical models and devices." In *3D Printing in Medicine: A Practical Guide for Medical Professionals*, edited by Frank J. Rybicki and Gerald T. Grant, pp. 97–111. Cham: Springer International Publishing, 2017. https://doi.org/10.1007/978-3-319-61924-8_10.

[18] Mitsouras, Dimitrios, Elizabeth George, Frank J. Rybicki. "Quality and safety of 3D-printed medical models." In *3D Printing in Medicine: A Practical Guide for Medical Professionals*, edited by Frank J. Rybicki and Gerald T. Grant, pp. 113–23. Cham: Springer International Publishing, 2017. https://doi.org/10.1007/978-3-319-61924-8_11.

Zbigniew Nawrat

6 Virtual operating theater for planning Robin Heart robot operation

6.1 Introduction

Virtual reality (VR), artificial reality, cyberspace, and augmented reality are the new languages of communication. The ability to use it allows you to transfer information to the previously unavailable level: multidisciplinary but specific, local and personalized but global and based on knowledge (artificial intelligence, big data analysis), spatial and physical, fictional and real, and pictorial and interactive. Let's learn this new language, a new method of communication, to shorten the learning curve; plan the treatment, taking into account all patient data and prospective knowledge; and provide the necessary information during surgery, in short, to reduce the number of medical errors.

6.2 Introduction to surgical operation

Surgery is a specific type of medical activity, assuming the use of direct physical methods of intervention, in a place damaged by illness or injury. Surgical operations and management system are a type of medical activity that is used to diagnose, prevent, and treat a patient.

Division due to objective and outcome of the operation includes the following:

1. An exploratory surgery, also called diagnostic, is aimed at diagnosing the disease.
2. Radical surgery, also called radical dissection, is a procedure aimed at complete cure of the disease (often excision of a part of a single organ).
3. Palliative surgery, also called alleviating, only improves the patient's condition, not removing the proper cause.
4. Plastic surgery changes the appearance or function of the organ.

The complexity of action is based on the need to assess the initial state (diagnosis) and to make decisions about the action spread over time and the roles of members of a special team.

The operation is a part of the patient's treatment strategy. The full treatment plan also includes the adoption of an appropriate method of rehabilitation and the planning of subsequent operations (including the preparation of the operation area for reoperation).

The planning of the operation includes defining the space and the object of the operation, the choice of methods, the materials and devices, the use of the operating and accompanying team, and finally the selection of sequences of a series of tools activities on tissue and organs. It is necessary to locate and describe pathological part of the human body operation space first. Describing means providing information about location, geometric features, and physical properties of tissues. Next, the approach path through patient's body for tools should be selected and optimized.

Operation optimization refers to the time and place of the operation (personalized based on diagnostic and prognostic data), human team, materials, instrumentation, and costs. Surgical operation by the adopted strategy (goal setting) and tactics (implementation method) is described. The tactics provide a possible and effective approach to use resources (human and material ones, knowledge, and tools) to achieve objectives.

In the simplest form, a typical planning process can be divided into the following elements: analysis of the patient's condition; goals—defining what is the subject of our intervention, what is the task to do; and strategy—defining how the goal can be achieved.

Tactics are the details of the strategy, precisely the specific actions and methods used during the performance of the task. Tasks and operations in surgery require the introduction of a specific impact (using physical, chemical, and biological phenomena) on biological tissues. A new area of surgical treatment is the corrective action on implantable elements (materials and devices). The strategy is modified by a constant flow of information during a surgical operation.

For surgery to be a planned process (standardization), it should have objective measurable features such as the following:

1. motion measurement (kinematics), physical (dynamics) and biological (e.g., by using biotechnological methods, stem cells, and cultured tissues) or chemical one;
2. assessment of the biological/physiological state before and after surgery;
3. economic evaluation (direct costs: materials and equipment; indirect costs: occupational and postoperative room occupancy; software/hardware costs: costs of using the IT network and maintaining telemedical readiness); and
4. staff activity (number, team members and time, and type of work).

The description of the work of the band resembles the recording of the theater scene—according to the scenario, actors written into the roles of action, choreography of people and tools (robots), language of communication, objects, division into acts, and a clear goal. It is not surprising that this place in the hospital is called the operational theater.

6.3 Modeling and planning of a surgical procedure

Modeling as a cognitive method plays a particularly important role in medical sciences, where the method of a physical experiment is difficult to implement because of the need to intervene in a living object (risk of losing health or life) and for ethical reasons [1].

Computer simulation methods and laboratory tests of physical models can be the basis for the preparation of surgical operations. The effectiveness of using robots in endovascular surgery largely depends on the optimization of design solutions for specific operations and proper planning of operations. The introduction of telemanipulators changes the perception [2] and, therefore, requires new training techniques to achieve the correct precision of the surgeon's work. Appropriate planning of the robot setting at the operating table, the correct location of the holes in the patient's body shells through which the tools with specific functionality and workspace will be inserted, provides the opportunity to perform a safe surgical procedure. The subject of planning is also a sequence of robot movements (choreography) and the selection of the right tools. The possibility of operating in the virtual space of the patient's body allows the surgeon to determine whether a given tool with defined geometric dimensions with defined degrees of freedom has the right range to perform the planned activities. VR technology is the perfect language for communication with surgeons and the field of testing innovative solutions.

In 1997, the team of the Foundation of Cardiac Surgery Development (Fundacja Rozwoju Kardiochirugrii im. Prof. Zbigniewa Religi [FRK]) led by the author started the first project in Poland (financed by the National Science Committee), a program of simulation of cardiac surgery procedures to optimize the operation effect.

The advisory system for the Robin Heart robot is currently being developed, available online during operations on the technical monitor of a control console. Adding physical features (e.g., blood flow and pressure) to the spatial objects (organ geometry) is a huge help in making decisions during surgery [1].

One of the pioneers of Polish robotics, Prof. A. Morecki, in a review [3] considers the following phase of robotic procedures:

1. Preoperative planning: the optimal strategy is defined based on the 3D computer model
2. Beginning of robot work: periodic robot calibration and telemanipulator operation in space with defined boundaries and areas of interest
3. Updating opinions and replanning: the robot starts working under the supervision of a doctor

The information (mainly the image) from the field of surgery allows us to confirm the compliance of the anatomy with expectations. If there is a deviation, the surgeon decides to change the strategy.

There are many publications proving the need of planning operations as a strategy deciding on the success of a surgery and a treatment process. Various management methodologies and their appropriate modifications are used. A detailed analysis of the operation requires the process to be divided into elements of the entire system (a surgeon, instruments, and a patient) with clearly defined evaluation parameters [4].

A very interesting analysis of operations and research on this subject can be found in the book edited by Dankelman et al. [5]. In the work of Kwon et al. [6], the sequences of 21 tasks, the so-called surgery task model of cholecystectomy, were obtained as a result of the analysis of recordings of six laparoscopic clinical operations. Research and analyses were conducted to optimize treatments. In the book of Gharagozloo and Najama [7], one can find a plan of almost all types of operations performed by the da Vinci robot. In Polish literature, it is worth paying attention to Marek Cisowski's postdoctoral dissertation describing selected cardiac surgeries [8], which is a summary of the performance of the Zeus robot as used for the first time in Katowice, Poland. The next interesting work in the field of general and colon robotic surgery (da Vinci robot) is from Wroclaw [9].

Outstanding works describing the technique of operations using the da Vinci robot are related to the activity of the student of Prof. Zbigniew Religa, Romuald Cichoń, at the clinic in Dresden (coauthor of many, commonly cited publications). Another pioneer of the surgery, Falk [10], clearly points out that progress depends on the introduction of new, functional tools; tissue stabilization techniques at the surgery site; and new methods of suturing, combining tissues, planning, and navigating computer tools. Falk [11] was the first to introduce and confirm the advantages of computer simulations and VR technologies and the so-called mixed reality (allows you to enter elements of real natural images) to plan coronary bypass surgery using the da Vinci robot.

It is worth noting that the main element of the management plan is a human—a surgeon. The studies of the ergonomics and biometrics of the surgeon's work are the basis for optimizing the way the surgery is carried out. Bernstein is regarded as one of the founders of the modern theory of human motor activity, and he included its foundations in his work on the structure of movements (1947). The beginning of the movement is, according to Bernstein, possible after imagining the goal and constructing the program of action. Movement of a human is based on keeping comparing the desired value with the current one regarding the indicators characterizing movement. Therefore, the motor coordination is "(...) overcoming the excessive number of degrees of freedom of the moving organism, that is, converting it into a controllable system" [12].

According to Bernstein, the information circulation time in an organism is 0.07–0.12 s. This is characterized by a frequency of 8–14 Hz, which is typical of the α wave of brain waves and muscle tremor. Movement coordination is the ability to perform complex movements accurately and quickly. The key role in the coordination of movements is played by the spatial orientation and kinesthetic skills of the differentiation of motion, based on sensory information. The introduction of robots and consoles as the operator's station changes the global system into a local one. The dexterity of the hand is important, not the movement of the whole body [1].

The possibilities of training conditional motor skills are unquestionable. Also in terms of motor skills coordination, there are great opportunities for improvement as a result of training impact. It has been shown that the learning curve, the time of reaching the appropriate efficiency, for robotic surgery is much faster than classic methods [13, 14].

Doctors expect rapid progress in the implementation of tools that are not only manipulative but also informative. During teleoperation, there is a problem of time shift between the movement and its image on the monitor. We are exploring the possibility of increasing the precision of operation by the appropriate formulation of a symbolic image associated spatially and an object related with the real image.

Surgery is also, and perhaps above all, a decision-making process. Making the right decisions is always a critical element of activity that involves the lack of full information from the past and uncertain future evaluation, as well as the lack of appropriate inference algorithms. Bernstein conceived biological "activity" or the ability of living organs to "anticipate" in such way. "The brain functions in two ways. It constructs the models of the past-present as well as stochastic extrapolations of these (models of the future). Any difference between the two not only constitutes a problem but also entails a probability distribution of its solution. This probability distribution will lead to the construction of a motor 'engram' (program)" [15]. Fact-based medicine and advisory programs greatly increase the likelihood of a doctor making the right "now" decisions to get the best solution for "tomorrow."

Let's try to analyze the decision-making process by the operator from the point of view of artificial intelligence methods used in process automation. This chapter contains a few basic definitions and discussions [16].

Decision-making situations can be divided into the following:

Determined (making decisions under conditions of certainty)

Random (in risk conditions)

Conflict (in conflict conditions, game theory)

In the decision-making process, the following phases can be distinguished:

Recognition (collection of information)

Modeling (construction of a decision-making model)

Deciding (choosing the best decision)

The implementation of the objective requires the use of available resources (material, financial, time, human, etc.) in the form of a strategy.

The surgeon often makes decisions in conditions of external uncertainty (lack of sufficient knowledge about the operating environment) and internal uncertainty (lack of knowledge and experience). The area of uncertainty can be reduced by using advisory and training systems and by planning using computer simulations and physical modeling [1].

The human decision-making process is based on one of two thought patterns:

1. Cartesian (cause-and-effect thinking based on classic logic, thinking precedes action, "I think ... so I decide")
2. Darwinian (trial and error method, action precedes decisions, "I check the effect of a decision") [16].

Robotic operators use both patterns. It is the surgeon, the operator, who decides about every move. According to the current rules, the robot cannot make the move itself. However, the time for autonomous robots is coming. For this kind of robotic surgery, planning will become the creation of a surgical robot task program. We can count on the rapid development of artificial intelligence and sensory devices necessary to achieve the right level of decision making based on the assessment of the space and the operation object. It will be a surgery based on facts obtained directly from the field of operations and analysis of databases, the so-called big data. The role of IT solutions is growing. According to R. Satava, a surgical robot today is more of an IT tool rather than a mechanical tool [17].

The principles of ergonomics should be applied when creating software—ensuring the effectiveness, efficiency, and satisfaction of the employee. These three properties describe software usability.

A surgical telemanipulator is a tool that must be adapted by the surgeon who controls it. Once we understand everything, we will be able to create independent surgical robots. Surgery will stop being an art and will become a science.

6.4 Training

Planning starts the process of preparing for a surgery. If the successful performance of surgical tasks requires the acquisition of new skills and their improvement, the appropriate training process should be implemented. In the past, the only way to know and control the patient's anatomical space, including the capture of pathological features associated with a given disease, was anatomical tests on the cadaver (or animal model). Currently, this role can be taken up to a virtual patient (anatomy) and a virtual operating room (operating room organization with tools and devices cooperating with surgeons at the operating table).

Introducing new surgical techniques moving the surgeon away from the operating table, like in teleoperations, introduces responsibility problems because of the risk of communication errors. To date, not all problems have been resolved. Ethical, practical, philosophical, and economic factors influence the development of remote control operation. The first evolution/revolution was associated with the introduction of endoscopic techniques, during which the surgeon's hands are only a few dozen centimeters away from the operation area. Currently, when we deal with the transmission of the signal, i.e., the will of the surgeon regarding the operation of the tools inside the patient's body in another city or on another planet, we must respond to new challenges (mastering physical phenomena and unknown technical solutions). Therefore, we need to develop research on the process of transmission of action, the effect of the work of a surgeon at a distance (optimization, i.e., adequate effectiveness with minimal risk). However, let's not forget about training. We also need to prepare the surgeon for this new type of profession. In surgery, training should include various technologies: (a) physical modeling, (b) VR, (c) manual training stands, and (d) computer stations. This story begins with the pelvitrainer recommended by Kurt Semm, a German surgeon and pioneer of endoscopic surgery. The pelvitrainer consists of a fiberglass box, single lens optic laparoscope, fiber optic light source, endoscopic camera, and video monitor. The first structured surgical training program in the United States (based on clinical service with subjective feedback from mentors [apprenticeship]) was created by Dr. William Halsted [18]. Currently, because of economic constraints, more attention was paid on the efficacy of surgical education [19].

The measurement of surgical efficiency is mainly related to the precision of movement and the implementation of mechanical (e.g., tying the knot or separation of tissue) and biological tasks (assessment of the patient's condition immediately after surgery, quality, and lifetime). The use of mini-invasive surgical methods has many advantages for the patient but is a technical challenge for the surgeon. Endoscopic tools deprive certain movement possibilities. The endoscopic tool is inserted into the patient's body through the hole (hereinafter referred to as the port), which is suitably reinforced as a type of ball joint during maneuvering the tool. On the one hand, the port plays the stabilizing role of this long tool during work; on the other hand, it limits the freedom of movement (reduces the number of degrees of freedom by 2) and changes the direction of the tool's movement opposite (left-right) to the movement of the hand holding the tool holder. A sense of touch the tissue is also changing. For the surgeon to be able to operate with the required precision in the conditions of reduced touch sensitivity (lack of force feedback) and space often presented on a two-dimensional monitor only (lack of sense of depth), it is necessary to acquire psychophysical skills during training exercises. A system of training devices for doctors to operate with the use of new developed mechatronic and robotic tools has been prepared in the Biocybernetics Lab of FRK [1, 20–26]. The photographs shown in Fig. 6.1 present good examples from the FRK history.

Medical simulations should be based on the geometrical representation of anatomy, soft tissue modeling (physics), and physiology. Currently, in most simulators, accurate haptic feedback is lacking—we have no connection between the deformability of the tissue and the physical interactions and feeling during the control of tool movements [27].

The training process of the medical team also requires a more natural, biological reality, which consists of the following:

a. Cadaver study
b. Animal preparation
c. Clinical experimental application

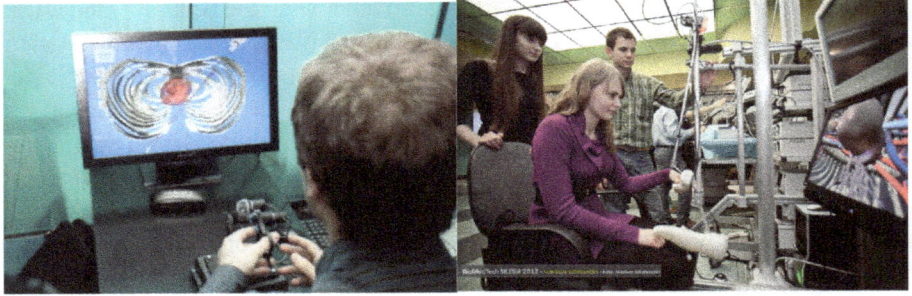

Virtual laparoscopic training station & Robin Heart Shell console with virtual robot [25].

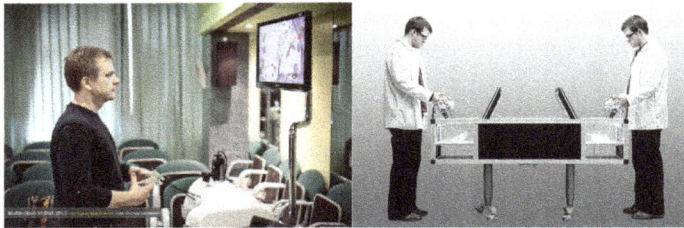

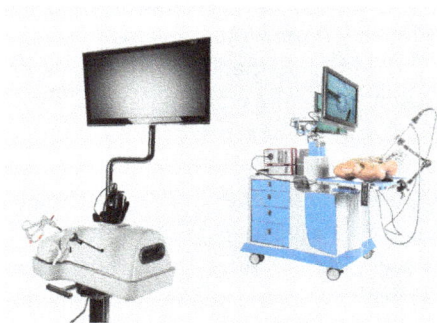

Classic laparoscopic training stations

Fig. 6.1: An original system of training stations prepared in the Biocybernetics Lab of FRK.

Training is the key to the success of future surgeons, but the learning curve, measured by the number of operations carried out to achieve the routine (time and effect of the operation), is much shorter for operations using telemanipulators. Currently, the importance of virtual space technology in training is growing because of the increasing reality of scenes and ease of access to launch training. The VR operating room, with Robin Heart robots, can be manipulated realistically with all of their functionality: an endoscope camera viewport displayed in a picture-in-picture technology; a human model with basic organs that might be exchanged to the ones from a patient

CT or NMR; and a surgery room with a surgery table, lamps, and all the basic equipment. The Robin Heart training system has been performed using EON software by the FRK team [20, 21].

6.5 Planning of robotic operations

Virtual surgery is a tool for the transparent visualization of an advanced surgical procedure. Using the VR technology, an interactive, fully controllable operating room model equipped with various Robin Heart surgical telemanipulators was made at the FRK.

Given the appropriate planning of the robot setting at the operating table, the correct location of the holes in the patient's body shells, through which the tools with specific functionality and workspace will be inserted, has a strong impact on the safe implementation of the surgical procedure. The subject of planning is also a sequence of robot movements (choreography) and the selection of the right tools. An important way to implement operations planning is to use virtual space technology. As a part of the Robin Heart project, the first virtual and robotic operating room in Poland was developed. The ability to operate in the virtual space of the patient's body allows the surgeon to determine whether a given tool with defined geometrical dimensions and certain degrees of freedom has the right range to perform the planned activities.

To prepare the robot well for the operation, it is necessary to know the principles of its operation. Robin Heart is a spherical robot with the appropriate range of permissible arm movement and the effective range of the tool inside the patient's body. The main assumption about the functionality of the Robin Heart telematic video kinematic chain is the construction of a double articulated quadrilateral to provide constant motion. The geometrical range and the mobility of the tool determine the potential operation space. The analysis of the impact of the tool selection and the location of the patient's intersection are the basis for surgery planning.

VR in the FRK in Zabrze is currently used in four extremely important and mutually related research areas:

1. as a training station for future surgeons, who can become familiar with the behavior of the model and way of controlling the Robin Heart robot,
2. as a tool for planning operational procedures with possible instruction in the course of proceedings,
3. as a tool to prepare the choreography of the robot (numerical set of information about the robot's position and all tools for various elements of the procedure) for the online consultancy program during the operation, and
4. as verification of the robot's design solutions based on their usefulness for a specific surgical procedure.

The VR room was equipped with all designed robots, mechatronic tools (Robin Heart Uni System), and selected typical surgical tools and elements of the operating room. VR technology can perfectly serve as an interactive training tool. The developed, among others, model of the FAMED operating table was controlled from the original or virtual remote control. The user has all structural cross sections to understand the operating principles and the ability to run specific device control functions. A laparoscopic surgery training set was made with position adjusters, which are physical holders of laparoscopic instruments. A robot training stand is prepared with the full features of a natural Robin Heart robot management position.

The original operating planning system allows saving selected sequences of images of robot and tool settings and a digital, unambiguous record of these settings in the coordinate system with respect to selected points on the patient's body, on the table, or on the operating room map. Images can be recalled on the consultant monitor of the Robin Heart Shell console. The recording of the coordinates of the robot's settings (settings of all the robot's degrees of freedom and its basis) will enable the reconstruction of the planned settings [1].

Figs. 6.2a–6.2d illustrate the planning of selected surgical procedures, mainly related to Robin Heart robotic animal experiments [1].

6.6 Robin Heart

The results of the project initiated by the author are the family of Robin Heart robots and the universal mechatronic tool series Robin Heart Uni System, which can be used during minimally invasive surgery on the heart and other soft tissues.

Robotics, as the technical discipline, deals with the synthesis of certain functions of the man by means of using some mechanisms, sensors, actuators, and computers. Among many types of robotics at present, one of the newest, but rapidly developed, is the branch of the medical robotics, which includes the manipulators and robots, dedicated to support surgery, therapy, prosthetics, and rehabilitation. Currently, several types of medical robotic systems have been applied in the surgery, including the following: robots replacing the assistant during the operation, such as Einstein, EndoAssist, or Polish prototype Robin Heart Vision, and surgical robots, such as da Vinci, Senhence, Versius, or Polish prototype Robin Heart (Fig. 6.3). The purpose of surgical robots is to improve efficiency and repeatability (standardization) and to reduce the invasiveness of surgical procedures (extension of the group of patients for whom successful surgical intervention is possible) [1].

The surgical robot has overcome the limitations of traditional endoscopic instruments that have only four degrees of freedom. Some of the robot's executive tools currently have 5–6 degrees of freedom and, additionally, some possibilities to perform complex, programmed movements. Robots have interchangeable tools used depending on the needs—harmonic knives, forceps, etc. The so-called quick connector should enable the quick replacement of the tool by the assistant

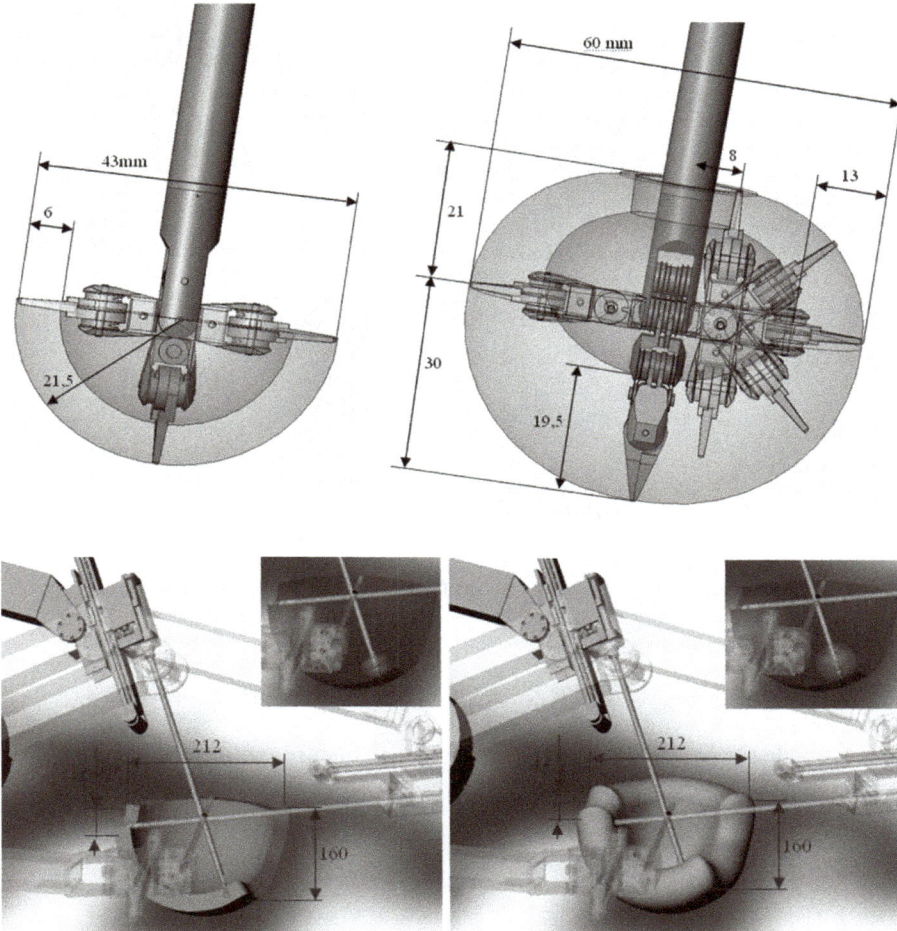

Fig. 6.2a: Working space for the Robin Heart tool with two and three rotary axes [1, 20, 21].

and ensure the possibility of sterile connection of the "clean" tool with the robot's fixed arm. The robot is a telemanipulator—a remote control device. The robot does not have to reflect the human's natural movements, but as a telemanipulator it is controlled.

The upper limb of a man fulfills two basic functions: (a) manipulative (manus—hand) performed by the hand with fingers and (b) extension arm performed by the arm with the forearm. The performed measurements (work space) and observations indicate that the surgeon works mainly by moving the wrist. The analysis of anatomy shows that wrist movements are possible in the range of –80° (palm flexion) and +70° (dorsal elevation) and in the perpendicular axis +20° and –20° (radial deviation). An ergonomic, appropriately designed motion detector, a haptic device, and a joystick play very important roles during precision telemanipulation.

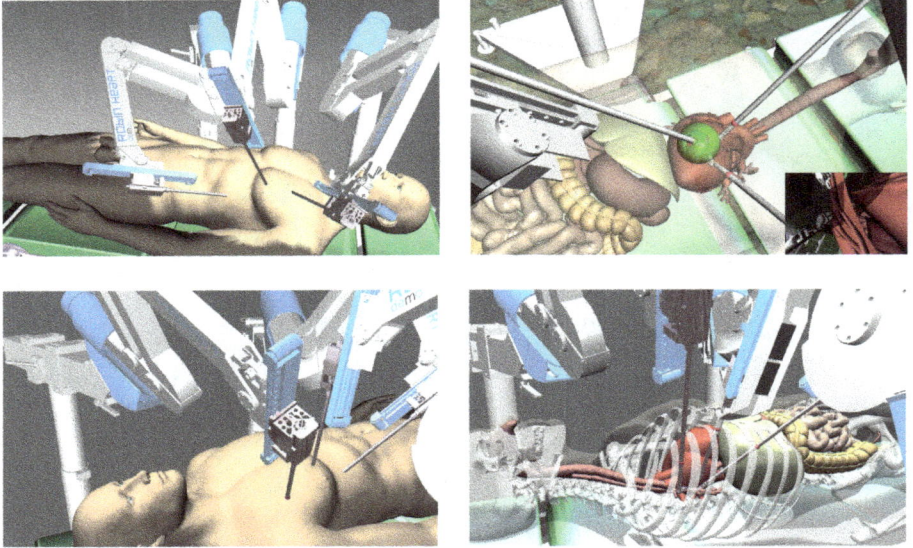

Fig. 6.2b: Operation planning for Robin Heart 1: (A) TECAB operation; (B) mitral valve surgery [1].

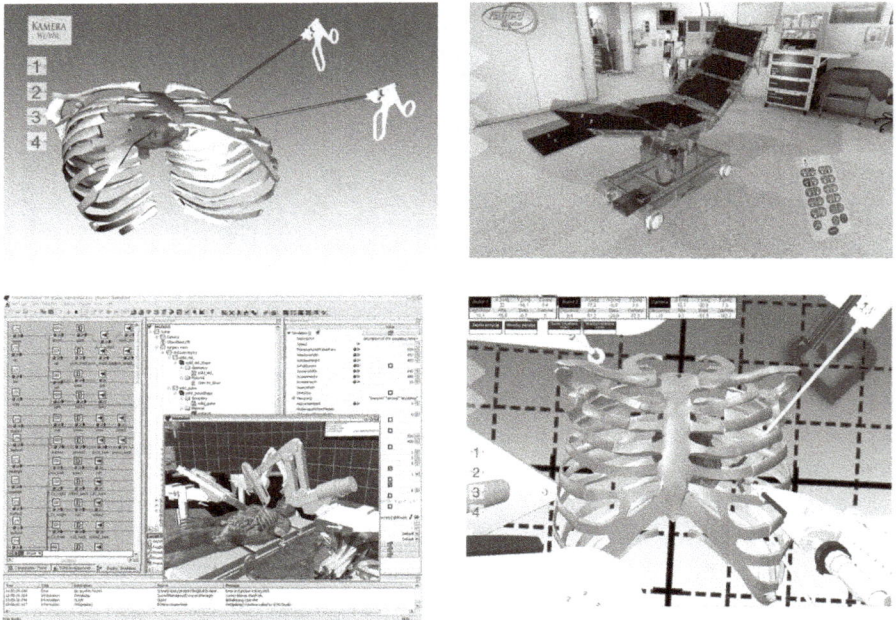

Fig. 6.2c: 3D model of laparoscopic tools, surgical table, and robot simulation made using EON Software by FRK [1, 22].

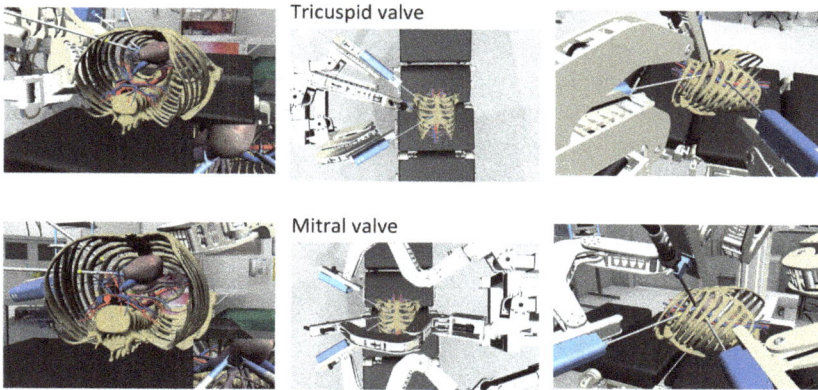

Fig. 6.2d: Example of planning the valve operation using the Robin Heart mc^2 robot [1].

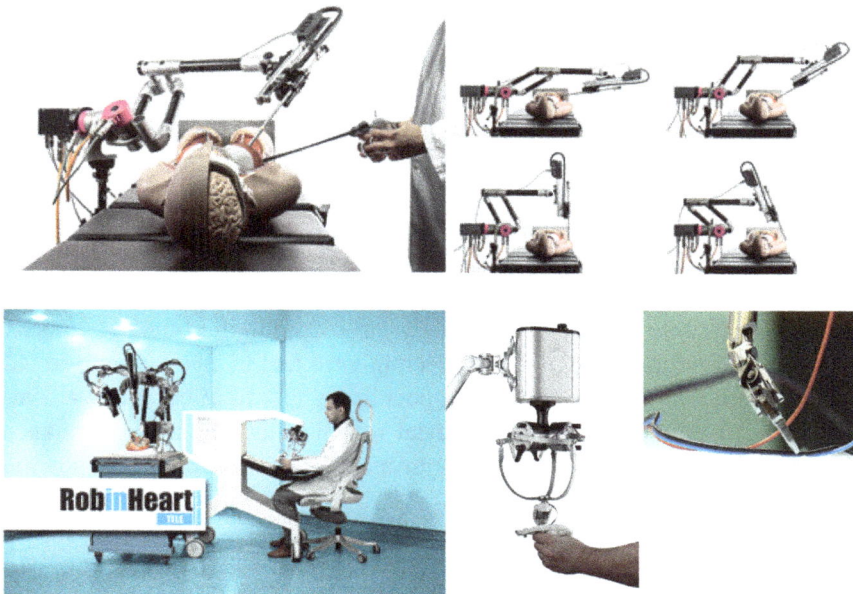

Fig. 6.3: Robin Heart PortVisionAble as a robot used to control the position of endoscope during laparoscopic operation and Robin Heart Tele as an example of surgical telemanipulator.

The Robin Heart Shell model constructed we constructed is an attempt to implement a natural mediator between the surgeon and the robot. A characteristic feature of the construction is its support on the operator's natural idea placed inside the operation space.

The process of projecting the Robin Heart robot starts by determining the tool-tissue reaction (the mechanical characteristic, the forces for specific operations, and the dynamic analysis of the work of a tool) and the person-tool/man-machine contact (kinematic analysis of the surgeon's motion). The surgeon's motion and the tool trajectory in a natural environment are analyzed with the use of optical biometry techniques. The forces applied during the impact of tools on tissue during typical surgical activities are measured. The construction assumptions as well as the functionality and ergonomics of the innovative tools can best be verified by means of video recording. As a result, a user-friendly surgical workstation (console) and an efficient surgical tool are constructed [1].

The robot, or rather a "telemanipulator" (which in its definition means that between the tool inside the patient's body and the surgeon's hand is the robotic arm and computer control system), is the first tool of the surgeon that allows support directly during work using the previously developed plans and advisory programs. It enables the introduction of a new standard in the surgeon's quality system.

The Robin Heart system (Figs. 6.3–6.5) includes a series of telemanipulators and automatic surgical tools as well as planning system, training system, and experts' program. The Robin Heart Shell console is equipped with a consulting program (online access on the screen) with patient's diagnostic information and picture/navigation data from operation planning. The 3D virtual operating theater introduced in our laboratory allows surgeons to train some elements of an operation and check the best placement of the ports.

In the Polish Robin Heart surgical robot, many of the original solutions were introduced: telescopic sliding motion to move the tool (2002), mechatronic tool "for the hand (2006) and the robot," and Robin Heart mc^2 (2010), which is the first surgical robot that can work for three persons (two surgeons and assistant responsible for endoscope orientation). The tool platform was modified in the TeleRobin project (2010). Robots and mechatronic tool have been in vitro and in vivo (animal) tested (Fig. 7). The Robin Heart family of Polish robots has a chance of becoming a commonly used high-tech technical and telemedical system facilitating the performance of some parts of operations in a minimally invasive, precise manner, safe for the patient and the surgeon [1].

6.7 Exercises with students

This chapter shows the proposal of exercises with students for "robotic surgery and virtual reality."

1. The use of robots and endoscopic tools introduces the elements of mechanics and limitations that are best understood by means of exercises during which we try to operate, gradually limiting the mobility in the next operator joints.

   Do you like detective stories, books, and crime movies? Imagine, therefore, that you only know the end of each story, losing the pleasure of seeking a solution. Hence, you are like customers who get a finished product. Scientific work has all the attributes of this joy of searching for the right answers. In the education process, we should recreate

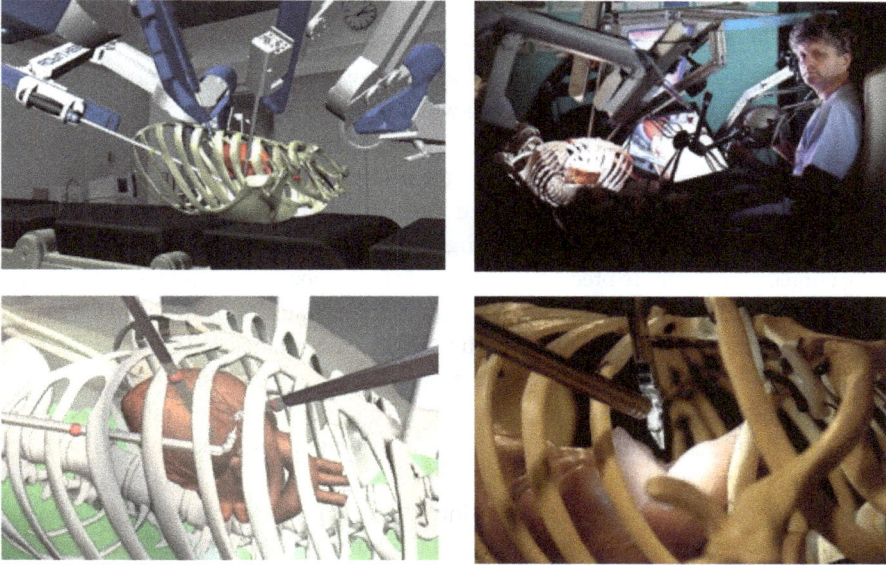

Fig. 6.4: Virtual and real conditions for testing the Robin Heart robot. The link between this type of modeling and computer-aided design (CAD) techniques is using an accurate CAD robot models in VR software together with a precise reflection of workspace geometry. This approach gives a surgeon easy and intuitive ways to understand technical information and use it to optimize and plan medical process [1, 24].

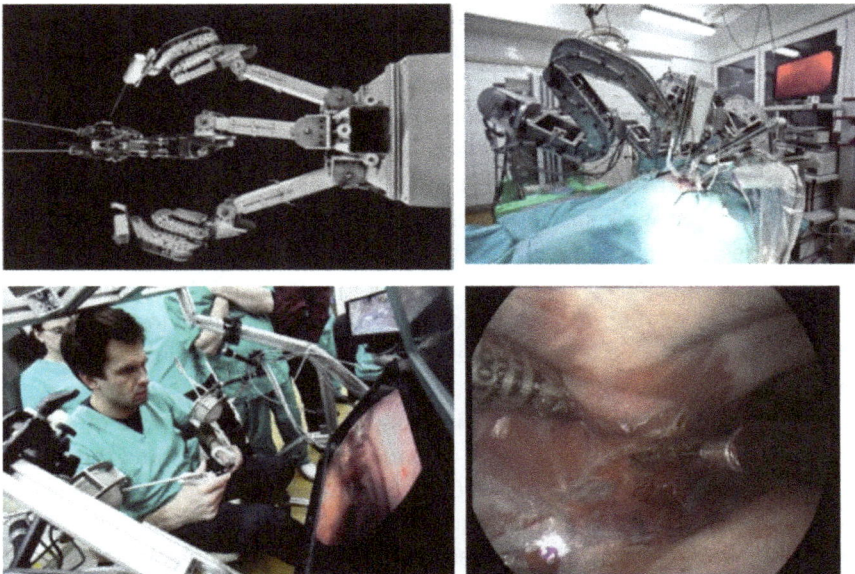

Fig. 6.5: Robin Heart mc² robot test during animal experiments [1].

for the students, although selected elements of the scientific work, to better understand the essence of the problem or the principle of operation of the device, which they get at their disposal. A good, simple, and easy example of such an approach is the modeling of movement limitations when using various surgical tools. To learn how to operate endoscopic tools or surgical robots, let us create a model of their work in limited mobility of the locomotor system of student. Let's put on the elbow, then the wrist of the hand, then the selected finger-stiffening bands, limiting the movement, and let's try to perform basic surgical operations in such a situation. Surely, the surgeon will be more precise and adequate to the possibilities after such a lesson.

2. The use of robots and endoscopic tools introduces limitations in the observation of the operation space. The video path with the camera inserted through the hole in the body of the patient can create a flat 2D or 3D spatial image on a monitor or eyepiece (depending on the equipment). To understand the limitations of the sense of depth and the resulting danger, an attempt should be made to perform the surgery with a 2D and 3D image.

3. The use of robots and endoscopic tools introduces limitations in terms of sensing the impact of tools on tissues. To understand the limitations of lack of force feedback and the resulting threats, it is necessary to carry out experiments to perform a given task, a surgical task in the situation of having the ability but also the inability to feel the respond of tools when working on a physical or virtual model. The best proposition for such tests is the use of a robot control console in the version with and without force feedback during the performance of a surgical task.

4. The use of robots—telemanipulators—introduces time delays in observing the effect of the tool during work. The best training and research station for the impact of information delay on the ability to perform precise operations is the use of a robot control console, predefined using an appropriate software with a different level of delay of the currently displayed image on the monitor.

5. Virtual operating room—exercises from the organization of an operation field. It is necessary to arrange the robots and decide on the location of the passage through the body shells of the patient (ports) in such a way that after choosing a tool with a given work space (associated with geometric dimensions and the number of degrees of freedom), it is possible to perform a specific operation such as heart or abdomen ones.

6. For the purpose of training the use of mechanical, mechatronic, and robotic endoscopic instruments, a virtual operating room with appropriate real handle can be used.

7. The use of robots—telemanipulators—introduces elements of the surgeon's ergonomics with the help of various types of motion units. To understand the role of the relationship between your haptic tool and the precision of the task, a series of experiments using a computer equipped with various drivers, mouse and joystick, can be performed. The simplest task can be, for example, the passage of the labyrinth with the help of various motion units.

All such possibilities, training stations, and research were developed and tested in the FRK in Zabrze (Fig. 6.6).

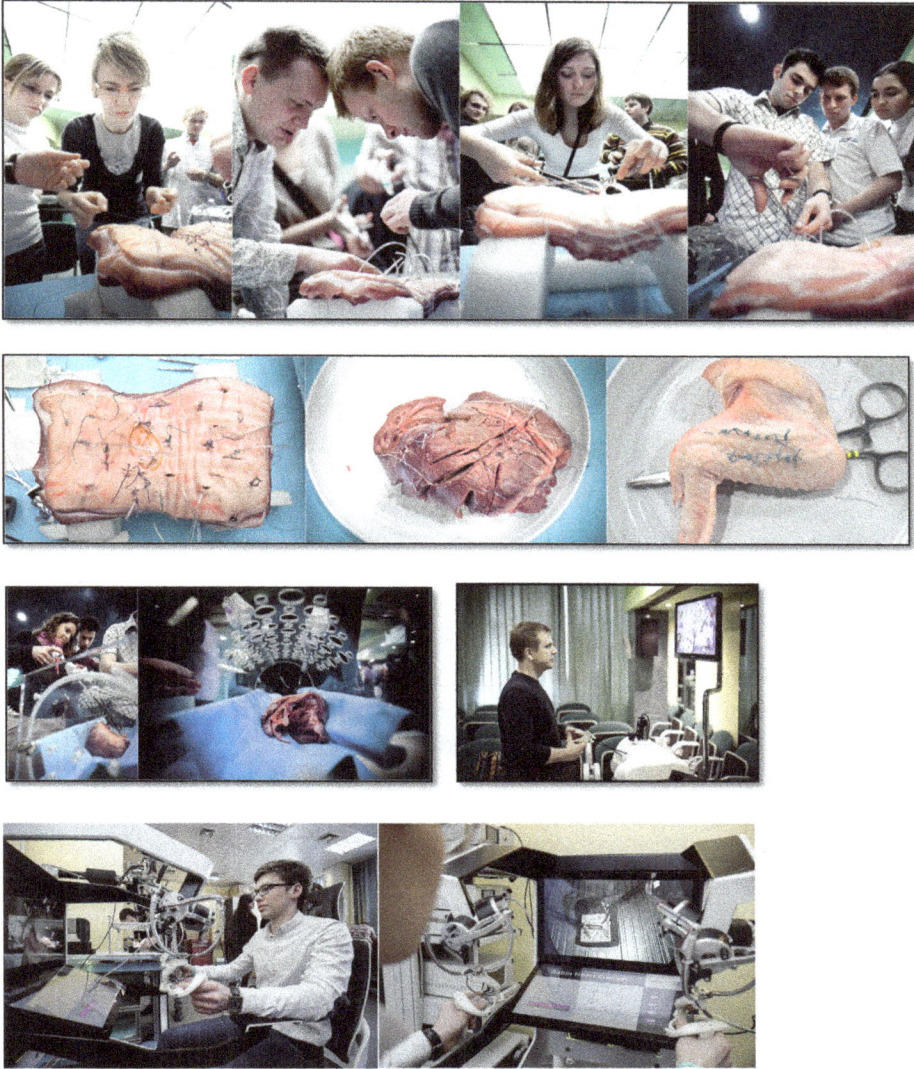

Fig. 6.6: Surgical workshop created by FRK & Medical University of Silesia. The principle of the workshops that have been going on for nearly 20 years is that participants start sewing on natural tissue, then use all training devices—from classic to laparoscopic to robotic ones. Both tests on natural tissue as well as plastic models are prepared (we have recently used fast 3D printing technology) and simulations in virtual space. Over 3,000 young people have participated in the free workshops in the FRK so far.

6.8 Summary

6.8.1 Robots and virtual space technologies

Robots have marked a breakthrough in many areas of modern science and life. They have already played an invaluable role in the development of manufacturing methods, and nowadays, they are entering the fields of medicine and education. Service robotics encourages the development of telemedical technologies used by patients and by medical staff. Surgical robots (new kind of tools) improve the quality and precision of surgical intervention and often reduce the invasiveness of operations.

Very important for current medicine education, VR technologies have been initiated by Ivan Sutherland who proposed the concept of "virtual worlds," giving an illusion of being present in a three-dimensional space created by means of a computer. In 1968, he demonstrated his "headband," which was a kind of helmet with screens in front of the eyes [22]. One of the best VR applications is for people with disabilities (simulation of lost physical activity in quasi-natural conditions). The modeling of behaviors in various situations in the therapy process of various phobias will also be used.

The implementation of VR techniques and stereoscopic imaging into telemedical systems requires certain conditions to be fulfilled by users. Beside a PC with an installed browser, users need stereoscopic glasses (to be able to see the image in 3D). The benefits involve, first, access to a lot of information transmitted in an understandable way in comparison with traditional methods of imaging and communication. Users have an opportunity of experiencing virtual operating theaters and tools used during operations, together with their technical description. They have a chance of controlling a cardiosurgical robot, of getting acquainted with the construction and mode of operation of different surgical tools and medical devices. Nevertheless, the most important quality of the VR technology is its interactivity, i.e., the possibility of involving participants in the space offered by the software and the inception of some physical features concerning the objects and the laws that govern their operation. It is possible to introduce "real" objects into virtual space [22].

The first applications of virtual space technology in Poland were related to medicine. FRK conducted pioneering works in Poland in the field of using virtual space technology in medicine. We were the first to buy software (EON) enabling the creation of an interactive operating room to be able to plan and train the use of new tools—surgical robots. We have introduced the solution in the form of a virtual operating theater to the educational package of implementing the Polish Robin Heart robot and to academic education.

Virtual surgery is a tool for the transparent visualization of an advanced surgical procedure. Using the VR technology, an interactive, fully controllable operating room model equipped with various Robin Heart surgical telemanipulators was made at the FRK. VR technology is the perfect language for communication with surgeons and the field of testing innovative solutions.

A proper development of surgeon skills requires joint work, through the use of both computer (including virtual) systems and tests on physical or hybrid models (with the elements of natural tissues). Tests with real tissues allow to the get to know properties of the natural object of the operation, what means to understand the crucial points of tool-tissue interaction. The essence of this abilities, so-called "the surgeon experience" (it is the most important factor of successful operation according to well-known literature), consists of the suitable relationship between a spatial imagination, manual efficiency, and medical knowledge and the abilities of taking quickly proper decisions connected with next stages of the executed procedure. This thing, which cannot be taught, is called "the talent," and it is the property reserved not for everyone. Medicine still tends to be an art despite more and more modern tools [27].

However, the use of virtual space technology has introduced a completely new quality: manipulation space enriched with information—real images, diagnostic + scientific data and imagination. The use of solutions based on the technology of virtual space has already changed the education of doctors, and now it is entering the operating rooms, supporting doctors in making decisions and increasing the chance of precision based on facts.

The surgeon, who usually works with limited access to information because many parts of the body are simply invisible, now obtains new possibilities, thanks to the enriched technology (augmented reality). This will bring a new quality of medical activity and measurable opportunities for patients.

The educational possibilities offered by virtual technologies are very important in areas inaccessible for testing because of ethical (medicine) or physical (space exploration) reasons. On the grounds of our experience, we claim that VR technologies constitute an excellent communication language to be used by engineers and physicians in the process of designing new surgical tools and robots.

A good choice of technologies required for the educational process is a standard that should be followed, even at the expense of teachers being replaced by avatars in some cases.

The future of the development of virtual space technologies in medicine depends on the implementation of new, ergonomic, and technical solutions. Soon, the introduction of the 5G networks will reduce the delay in sending high-resolution images. This means that the use of telemanipulators (at a distance of 100 km or more) will be more common—especially in the fields of consultancy, rehabilitation, and treatment tasks. Physical limitations remain because the speed of light or the transmission of information is limited. This means that in the category of cosmic medicine—e.g., related to the care of people traveling to Mars—we need to find other solutions. The development of artificial intelligence, sensory, and VR technologies will soon allow the robots to become independent. There are now completely new devices on the market that allow introducing the possibility of using augmented reality in real time. Perhaps the breakthrough will be Microsoft's introduction of the HoloLens 2 system with spatial anchors (will allow to share holograms with others via the Internet) and remote rendering (it will allow direct streaming of holograms in high quality to 100 million polygons).

Today, new technological equipment allows you to present spatial images on monitors, screens, or glasses, adding real elements. More and more companies are introducing professional applications of even a smartphone in medical practice to education, planning, and medical measurements. However, new developments in the form of presentation methods combined with measurements online and advanced medical data analysis (artificial intelligence) will be the future. In many academic centers, virtual technology has been introduced into the scope of training, and we also have several world-class Polish companies creating applications implemented clinically (Fig. 6.7). In this way, engineers help reduce the area of uncertainty that accompanies decision making during a doctors' work. They increase the effectiveness of medical actions undertaken, and they cocreate new medical standards. This future has already come.

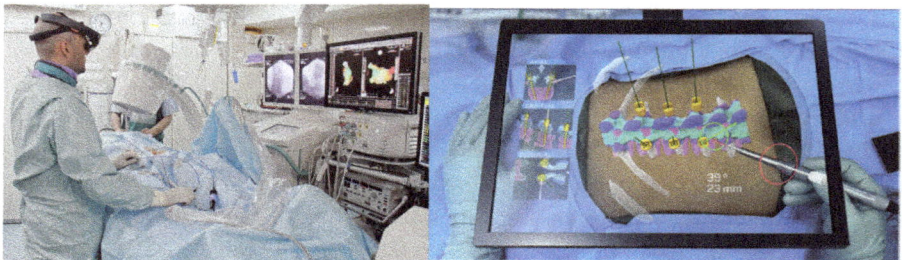

Fig. 6.7: (Right) In May 2017, an ablation of the base of an atrial fibrillation was performed in the electrophysiology workshop of the cardiology clinic at the Medical University of Warsaw (as a permanent treatment for cardiac arrhythmia), during which medical personnel in Poland were presented for the first time with the capabilities of the Carna Life analytical telemedicine system (https://medapp.pl/projekty-rd/projekt-holo/). (Left) HoloSurgical Inc., a digital surgery company, announced in 2019 a successful first in human surgical procedure utilizing the ARAI™, an augmented reality and artificial intelligence-based surgical navigation system, with 3D anatomical visualization for presurgical planning, real-time intraoperative guidance, and postsurgical data analytics (https://www.newgenapps.com/blog/5-incredible-uses-of-virtual-reality-in-medicine).

6.9 References

[1] Nawrat Z. *Robot chirurgiczny—projekty, prototypy, badania, perspektywy. Rozprawa habitacyjna*. Katowice, 2011.

[2] Shimoga KB, Khosla PK. "Touch and force reflection for telepresence surgery." *Proceedings of the IEEE Engineering in Medicine and Biology Society (EMBS)*, pp. 1049–1050. Baltimore, 1994.

[3] Morecki A. Medical robots selected problem. *Biocybernetics and Biomedical Engineering* 20, no. 3 (2000): 109–30.

[4] Boer KT, Gouma DJ, Grimbergen CA, Dankelman J. "Evaluation of the surgical process." *Engineering for Patient Safety Issue in Minimally Invasive Procedures*. Edited by Dankelman J, Grimbergen CA, Stassen HG, Mahwah, NJ: Lawrence Erlbaum Associates, 2005.

[5] Dankelman J, Grimbergen CA, Stassen HG. *Engineering for Patent Safety. Issues in Minimally Invasive Procedures*. London: Lawrence Erlbaum Associates, 2005.

[6] Kwon DS, Ko SY, Kim J. "Intelligent laparoscopic assistant robot through surgery task model: how to give intelligence to medical robots." In *Medical Robotics*. Edited by Bozovic V. Vienna: I-Tech, 2008.

[7] Gharagozloo F, Najam F. *Robotic Surgery*. The McGraw-Hill Companies, 2009.

[8] Cisowski M. "Miniinwazyjne pomostowanie gałęzi międzykomorowej przedniej lewej tętnicy wieńcowej z wykorzystaniem techniki wideoskopowej. *Rozprawa habilitacyjna.*" *Annales Academiae Medicae Silesiensis* Supl. 69 (2004).

[9] Zawadzki M, Krzystek-Korpacka M, Rząca M, Czarnecki R, Obuszko Z, Witkiewicz W. "Introduction of robotic surgery into a community hospital setting: a prospective comparison of robotic and open colorectal resection for cancer." *Digestive Surgery* 34, no. 6 (2017): S489–94.

[10] Falk V, Diegeler A, Walther T, Banusch J, Brucerius J, Raumans J, Autschbach R, Mohr FW. "Total endoscopic computer enhanced coronary artery bypass grafting." *European Journal of Cardio-Thoracic Surgery* 17 (2000): 38–4.

[11] Falk V, Mourgues F, Adhami L, Jacobs S, Thiele H, Nitzsche S, Mohr FW, Coste-Maniere E. "Cardio navigation: planning, simulation, and augmented reality in robotic assisted endoscopic bypass grafting." *Annals of Thoracic Surgery* 79 (2005): 2040–7.

[12] Rynkiewicz T. *Struktura zdolności motorycznych oraz jej globalne i lokalne przejawy*. AWF w Poznaniu. Poznań, 2003.

[13] Dakin G, Gagner M. "Comparison of laparoscopic skills performance between standard instruments and two surgical robotic systems." *Surgical Endoscopy* 17 (2003): 574–9.

[14] Seibold U, Kübler B, Hirzinger G. "Prototype of instrument for minimally invasive surgery with 6-axis force sensing capability." *Proceedings of the IEEE International Conference on Robotics and Automation*, pp. 498–503. Barcelona, Spain, March 18–20, 2005.

[15] Bongaardt R, Meijer OG. "Bernstein's theory of movement behavior: historical development and contemporary relevance." *Journal of Motor Behavior* 32, no. 1 (April 2000): 57–71.

[16] Bukowski LA. *Wybrane problemy automatyzacji złożonych problemów decyzyjnych. Metody sztucznej inteligencji w automatyzacji procesów. Red*, pp. 19–30. Edited by Bukowski LA. Kraków: Akapit, 2000.

[17] Satava RM. "Surgery 2001: a technologic framework for the future." Surgical Endoscopy 7 (1993): 111–3.

[18] Halsted WS. "The training of the surgeon." *Johns Hopkins Hospital Bulletin* 15 (1904): 267–75.

[19] Debas HT. "Impact of managed care on funding of surgical residencies." Archives of Surgery 130 (1995): 929–30.

[20] Nawra Z, Koźlak M. "Modelowanie I testowanie robota Robin Heart wykorzystując technologie przestrzeni wirtualnej." In *Postepy Technologii Biomedycznych 1/Advances in Biomedical Technology 1*, pp. 135–46. Edited by Zbigniew Nawrat, 2007.

[21] Nawrat Z, Kozlak M. "Robin Heart system modeling and training in virtual reality." *Journal of Automation, Mobile Robots and Intelligent Systems* 1, no. 2 (2007): 62–6.

[22] Nawrat Z, Sadowski W. "Standard and technologies. Opportunities—virtual reality technology." In *E-enjoy ICT Quality Book*, pp. 103–4. Edited by Zbigniew Nawrat, 2010.

[23] Nawrat Z, Koźlak M. "Possibilities of virtual reality technology application for education and surgeon training." In *Medical Robots 1*, pp. 125–34. Edited by Zbigniew Nawrat, 2010.

[24] Nawrat Z. "Case study. Tele-Student—deliberations on effective education of medical students." In *E-enjoy ICT Quality Book*, pp. 83–9. Edited by Zbigniew Nawrat, 2010.

[25] Małota Z, Nawrat Z, Sadowski W. "Minimally invasive surgery simulation." *Engineering of Biomaterials* XVII, no. 126(2014): 2–11.

[26] Malota Z, Nawrat Z, Sadowski W. "Benchmarking for surgery simulators." In *Soft and Stiffness-Controllable Robotics Solutions for Minimally Invasive Surgery: The STIFF-FLOP Approach*, pp. 309–32. Edited by Jelizaveta Konstantinova, Helge Wurdemann, Ali Shafti, Ali Shiva, and Kaspar Althoefer. River Publishers Series in Automation, Control and Robotics, 2018.

[27] Nawrat Z, Kostka P, Koźlak M, Małota Z, Dybka W, Rohr K, Sadowski W. "Innovative technology application for education and surgeon training." In *Postepy Technologii Biomedycznych 2/ Advances in Biomedical Technology 2*, pp. 173–81. Edited by Zbigniew Nawrat, 2008.

Piotr Mazur, Maciej Bochenek, Krzysztof Bartuś, Roman Przybylski, and Bogusław Kapelak

7 Hybrid room: Role in modern adult cardiac surgery

7.1 Introduction

A hybrid approach was initially proposed in the 1990s, as a combination of means available only in the catheterization laboratory with those typical for the operating room. The aim was to decrease the procedure invasiveness, while expanding the spectrum of cardiovascular lesions that could be tackled [1]. Angelini and colleagues [2] presented the first case series comprising six individuals submitted to an integrated surgical and percutaneous approach (minimally invasive direct coronary artery bypass [MIDCAB] with left internal mammary artery [LIMA] graft to the left anterior descending [LAD] artery with multivessel percutaneous coronary intervention [PCI] to non-LAD vessels), followed by a report of 18 cases in 1999 [3]. Today, hybrid procedures are performed routinely by dedicated teams, consisting of cardiac and/or vascular surgeons, along with invasive and noninvasive cardiologists or radiologists, supported by anesthesiologists and perfusionists, nurses, and technicians. The workplace for such a broad group of specialists and a manifestation of multidisciplinary approach toward patient care is a hybrid room.

The growing application of endovascular procedures and the complex minimally invasive cardiac and vascular surgeries lead to increasing imaging requirements in the operating room. Mobile image intensifier systems (C-arms) are often limited in terms of their image quality, radiation safety, and overheating. On the other hand, catheterization laboratories are not suitable for performing complex procedures involving cardiopulmonary bypass (CPB). Not only do they fail to meet the space requirements, but also there is difficulty managing asepsis. Hybrid rooms are modern (usually large) operating theaters, which provide comfort and safety to the surgical team, optimal radiation management, and best compromise between imaging quality and asepsis.

7.2 Components of the hybrid room

7.2.1 Surgical requirements

As all operating theaters, hybrid rooms should comply with asepsis requirements, typical for procedures with open approaches and implantation of medical devices. Beside an operating table offering a wide range of spatial settings (operating table must be radiolucent and is often made of nonmetallic carbon fiber [4]) and proper shadeless overhead surgical light, a hybrid room is required to have atmosphere control to prevent infections [5]. Proper laminar airflow and positive room pressure should be considered at the time of hybrid room planning, and used materials should be chosen as to minimize the release of any airborne particles. The presence and availability of all crucial elements of a traditional operating room, including cautery knife, suction, surgical sutures, and instruments, is necessary for easy conversion from a minimally invasive or percutaneous procedure to a fully open approach. The latter requires a possibility to back off the imaging system quickly, which should be easily and intuitively maneuverable. For cardiac hybrid rooms, it is also necessary to have an operational CPB machine on standby, and a clinical perfusionist should be a constant member of the team.

7.2.2 Room requirements

A large team of physicians, technicians, and nurses works with a single patient. Spatial requirements are substantial, as the team can count up to 20 members; a hybrid room should have a large area ($\geq$70 m^2) to accommodate the personnel along with the equipment, including the fixed C-arm. Ceiling-mounted monitors should be abundantly present to allow all team members to visualize the images simultaneously (including, for example, angiographic and echocardiographic images together with hemodynamic monitoring [6]).

7.2.3 Fixed C-arm and imaging techniques

Hybrid rooms should offer good imaging quality resulting from the use of fixed high-quality radiological equipment. A basic imaging modality in the hybrid room is fluoroscopy, offering a live 2D x-ray view of progressing medical devices within the body. In cardiac interventions, quality requirements are high, and the fixed C-arm should be able to deliver a fluoroscopy with a high frame rate. Fixed C-arms are usually mounted to the ceiling or the floor, most of them having the ability to be moved away when not in use. Image quality improves, as image intensifiers are replaced by flat panel detectors. These offer a higher signal-to-noise ratio, have a wider dynamic signal range, and reduce the geometric distortion [5]. Other modalities (like integrated ultrasound, electromagnetic navigation systems, etc.) can be incorporated into the system. Moreover, advanced digital image processing methods are implemented to meet the needs of specific clinical situations, such as valve deployment planning during TAVI. A 3D C-arm CT can be obtained quickly to assist valve replacement or aortic stent graft placement. Workstations that allow image postprocessing are crucial for any hybrid room, as they not only allow planning and guidance but also support immediate intraoperative assessment of complex cases, e.g., intraoperative vessel analysis using automated vessel analyzing software to accurately size the implantable device.

All imaging devices within the hybrid room should be integrated into the institutional network to easily exchange information with other imaging modalities, and a connection with Picture Archiving and Communication Systems is mandatory. In addition, the control area for radiological technicians should have a direct view of the surgical field.

7.2.4 Image fusion

Live fluoroscopy imaging can be enriched by a superimposition of a 3D model of the vasculature, obtained preoperatively (CT or MRI) or periprocedurally (contrast-enhanced cone-beam CT). Original idea of simple approximate superimposition of 3D volume rendering on the vasculature evolves into more complex models, integrating case-specific information chosen by the operators, such as vessels ostia, best gantry angulation to support catheterization of those vessels, etc. This has been used in complex endovascular aneurysm repair with branched grafts [6]. The future of hybrid rooms will likely be influenced by the emergence of augmented reality technologies. Possible solutions that could find application include projection of data extracted from preoperative imaging studies on live fluoroscopy, or directly on patient skin, and virtual representations of x-ray exposure within the room. The new generation of image fusion will not only make the operator feel safer and more comfortable but also improve safety and efficiency of the hybrid room.

7.2.5 Radiation safety

Hybrid rooms with fixed imaging systems generally deliver less radiation than mobile C-arms; however, any personnel operating within this environment should use personal protection and radiation dosimeters, following the "as low as reasonably achievable" principles. Also, the room design itself is different from traditional operating rooms, including lead-lined walls and doors to reduce radiation outside the room, clear shields mounted to the ceiling (to be placed between the patient and the operator), lead aprons, etc. The building design needs to consider these requirements when planning a hybrid room.

7.2.6 Training

A growing number of hybrid procedures are performed worldwide, and this has implications for both interventionalists and surgeons. Vascular surgeons adopted percutaneous approach early, whereas cardiac surgeons were rarely trained in endovascular skills. The need for cross training is essential for multidisciplinary approach, and surgeons should be trained in the catheterization laboratory before moving to the hybrid room. Conversely, cardiologists and interventional radiologists should gain exposure to proper surgical technique and knowledge on anatomy. Although "hybrid specialists" are emerging, the role of the Heart Team is not to be underestimated and still vital.

7.3 Clinical application of the hybrid room

7.3.1 TAVI

TAVI has been performed since 2002, when Alain Cribier performed the first implantation in human [7]. Since that transfemoral implantation of a pericardial valvular prosthesis under fluoroscopic guidance, tremendous progress has been done. Currently, TAVI is the procedure of choice in patients deemed to have to high a surgical risk and plays an important role in valvular disease treatment. In some countries, TAVI represents almost half of interventions on the aortic valve [8], and the number of implantations has long exceeded 100000 [9]. Valve bioprostheses undergo crimping to minimize their size and represent grossly three main types:
- Balloon-expandable devices; e.g., Sapien valve (Edwards Lifesciences, Irvine, CA)
- Self-expanding devices; e.g., Evolut valve (Medtronic, Minneapolis, MN)
- Mechanically expandable devices; e.g., Lotus valve (Boston Scientific, Marlborough, MA)

The approaches used in TAVI include percutaneous transfemoral implantation, transapical implantation through small left lateral thoracotomy, or transaortic implantation, the latter usually requiring sternotomy. A dedicated Heart Team, always including a cardiac surgeon, should perform any such procedure. Although percutaneous transfemoral TAVI can be performed in either an interventional cardiology suite or a hybrid room (size of implantation systems is decreasing), the remaining types of procedures are best suited for hybrid rooms because of a larger surgical component. Procedural invasiveness gradually decreases, with straightforward transfemoral cases being performed under local anesthesia. A recent study of 12121 TAVI procedures performed in 48 French centers showed similar midterm mortality after TAVI performed in catheterization laboratory and in a hybrid room [10]. Notwithstanding, a cardiac hybrid room is best suited for the treatment of complications (such as vascular injury, myocardial perforation, or valve migration), where emergency conversion to a fully open approach with CPB use is possible immediately. Other possible approaches, such as transiliac, transaxillary, or transcarotid, are used less frequently.

New devices are vigorously developed, and the market is expanding because of excellent TAVI results. The PARTNER trials showed that TAVI was superior to medical therapy in inoperable patients (cohort B [11]) and had similar results to surgery in high-risk patients (cohort A [12]). Recent PARTNER 3 trial showed TAVI noninferiority compared with surgery in low-risk subjects for balloon-expandable devices [13], whereas Evolut low-risk trial presented similar results for self-expandable prostheses [14]. The trial data should be interpreted cautiously and still need to be verified by registries and real-life data; however, TAVI has already gained a great popularity. Despite that, the number of classic surgeries did not drop dramatically [8]. The undebatable advantage of TAVI is that it can be practiced on computerized phantoms, a feature unavailable for surgeons. Also, a growing body of evidence supports the notion that TAVI might be helpful in patients with previous surgeries (e.g., patient with a history of coronary artery bypass grafting [CABG] who developed aortic stenosis) or those who suffer from prosthetic dysfunction (valve-in-valve procedures) [6]. One should bear in mind, however, that infectious complications of prosthetic valve implantations (infectious endocarditis) are always managed surgically, irrespectively of the initial implantation technique. Hybrid interventions on other valves are currently under development, with mitral valve implantation being the most advanced.

7.3.2 Hybrid coronary artery revascularization

Hybrid coronary artery revascularization combines surgical technique with percutaneous interventions for multivessel coronary artery disease in a structured fashion. Usually, off-pump MIDCAB of the LAD is done through a small left lateral thoracotomy, whereas PCI-remaining non-LAD lesions are addressed with PCI. This approach is suitable for individuals who present with a high-grade multivessel coronary disease, whose LAD lesion is proximal whereas the peripheral vessel is surgically available, and the remaining lesions are suitable for PCI [1], especially in the setting of lacking graft material or LAD anatomy unfavorable for PCI. Hybrid coronary revascularization bases on the concept that LIMA to LAD graft is the main source of benefit from CABG, as LIMA-LAD grafts are known to have excellent long term patency (>95% after 20 years [15]). Hence, the arguable benefit of CABG is sustained by performing minimally invasive LIMA-LAD grafting, whereas other vessels are treated percutaneously [6]. Typically, MIDCAB is done first to provide protection of LAD territory during PCI and to prevent exposure to dual antiplatelet therapy during surgery [6]. It can be a one- or two-stage procedure, yet the perfect procedural timing is still to be established. In case of one-stage procedures performed in a hybrid room, the revascularization is complete with minimal patient discomfort [1]. Furthermore, the performance of the LIMA-LAD anastomosis can be immediately verified angiographically. CABG may also be combined with concomitant carotid artery stenting, whereas PCI can be a part of a hybrid procedure involving valve replacement, which can be done minimally invasive with less risk in such setting.

7.3.3 Endovascular aortic repair

Endovascular aortic repair is one of the most common procedures performed in hybrid rooms, especially if the indication is aortic aneurysm. Open repair of thoracoabdominal aortic aneurysms carries a high morbidity and mortality and was essentially replaced by endovascular techniques in cases with suitable anatomy. Hybrid room also finds increasing application in the treatment of Stanford type A acute aortic dissections, enabling exact diagnosis of coronary status and downstream organ malperfusion [16]. The perioperative diagnostic possibilities the hybrid room has to offer can alter the plan of surgical attack and influence the design of surgical and endovascular treatment, remaining safe for the patients [16]. In hybrid rooms equipped with CT capabilities, the verification of stent graft placement and early detection and correction of endoleaks (which might remain undetected with classic fluoroscopy [17]) are possible, also facilitating placement of branched or fenestrated grafts.

7.3.4 Hybrid antiarrhythmic procedures

Atrial fibrillation (AF) affects a growing number of patients, and the treatment of choice in case of paroxysmal AF is catheter ablation, if pharmacotherapy fails. Despite the high success rate (approx. 80%), the recurrences are common, and multiple procedures are frequently required [18]. The surgical treatment of AF, based on the procedure proposed by Cox and colleagues (Cox-Maze procedure), where the pathological conduction pathways are transected [19], has excellent efficacy, at the cost of invasiveness. With the development of surgical ablation tools, Maze procedure can be performed thoracoscopically, in a minimally invasive fashion; nevertheless, the less invasive approaches often lack transmurality and are less efficacious than the actual atrial wall transection. Hybrid approach combines both transvenous endocardial and thoracoscopic epicardial ablation to maximize the effect. Furthermore, left atrial appendage (where thrombi in case of AF are frequently generated) can be occluded minimally invasive in the hybrid room).

7.4 Conclusions

Hybrid rooms have become a necessary part of any cardiovascular hospital, enabling a whole spectrum of procedures that would otherwise be unavailable. This evolutionary concept integrating advanced imaging modalities with safety of an operating theater offers new possibilities, also by bringing together diverse and multidisciplinary teams. In the near future, augmented reality is likely to enter the daily routine of many hybrid rooms.

7.5 References

[1] Papakonstantinou NA, Baikoussis NG, Dedeilias P, Argiriou M, Charitos C. "Cardiac surgery or interventional cardiology? Why not both? Let's go hybrid." *Journal of Cardiology* 69 (2017): 46–56.

[2] Angelini GD, Wilde P, Salerno TA, Bosco G, Calafiore AM. "Integrated left small thoracotomy and angioplasty for multivessel coronary artery revascularisation." *Lancet* 347 (1996): 757–8.

[3] Lloyd CT, Calafiore AM, Wilde P, Ascione R, Paloscia L, Monk CR, et al. "Integrated left anterior small thoracotomy and angioplasty for coronary artery revascularization." *Annals of Thoracic Surgery* 68 (1999): 908–11, discussion 11–2.

[4] Fillinger MF, Weaver JB. "Imaging equipment and techniques for optimal intraoperative imaging during endovascular interventions." *Seminars in Vascular Surgery* 12 (1999): 315–26.

[5] Hertault A, Sobocinski J, Spear R, Azzaoui R, Delloye M, Fabre D, et al. "What should we expect from the hybrid room?" *Journal of Cardiovascular Surgery* (Torino) 58 (2017): 264–69.

[6] Kaneko T, Davidson MJ. "Use of the hybrid operating room in cardiovascular medicine." *Circulation* 130 (2014): 910–7.

[7] Cribier A, Eltchaninoff H, Bash A, Borenstein N, Tron C, Bauer F, et al. "Percutaneous transcatheter implantation of an aortic valve prosthesis for calcific aortic stenosis: first human case description." *Circulation* 106 (2002): 3006–8.

[8] Beckmann A, Funkat AK, Lewandowski J, Frie M, Ernst M, Hekmat K, et al. "Cardiac surgery in Germany during 2014: a report on behalf of the German Society for Thoracic and Cardiovascular Surgery." Thoracic and Cardiovascular Surgeon 63 (2015): 258–69.

[9] Webb JG, Wood DA. "Current status of transcatheter aortic valve replacement." *Journal of the American College of Cardiology* 60 (2012): 483–92.

[10] Spaziano M, Lefevre T, Romano M, Eltchaninoff H, Leprince P, Motreff P, et al. "Transcatheter aortic valve replacement in the catheterization laboratory versus hybrid operating room: insights from the France TAVI Registry." *JACC Cardiovascular Interventions* 11 (2018): 2195–203.

[11] Leon MB, Smith CR, Mack M, Miller DC, Moses JW, Svensson LG, et al. "Transcatheter aortic-valve implantation for aortic stenosis in patients who cannot undergo surgery." *New England Journal of Medicine* 363 (2010): 1597–607.

[12] Smith CR, Leon MB, Mack MJ, Miller DC, Moses JW, Svensson LG, et al. "Transcatheter versus surgical aortic-valve replacement in high-risk patients." *New England Journal of Medicine* 364 (2011): 2187–98.

[13] Mack MJ, Leon MB, Thourani VH, Makkar R, Kodali SK, Russo M, et al. "Transcatheter aortic-valve replacement with a balloon-expandable valve in low-risk patients." *New England Journal of Medicine* 380 (2019): 1695–705.

[14] Popma JJ, Deeb GM, Yakubov SJ, Mumtaz M, Gada H, O'Hair D, et al. "Transcatheter aortic-valve replacement with a self-expanding valve in low-risk patients." *New England Journal of Medicine* 380 (2019): 1706–15.

[15] Tatoulis J, Buxton BF, Fuller JA. "Patencies of 2127 arterial to coronary conduits over 15 years." *Annals of Thoracic Surgery* 77 (2004): 93–101.

[16] Tsagakis K, Konorza T, Dohle DS, Kottenberg E, Buck T, Thielmann M, et al. "Hybrid operating room concept for combined diagnostics, intervention and surgery in acute type A dissection." *European Journal of Cardio-Thoracic Surgery* 43 (2013): 397–404.

[17] Biasi L, Ali T, Hinchliffe R, Morgan R, Loftus I, Thompson M. "Intraoperative DynaCT detection and immediate correction of a type Ia endoleak following endovascular repair of abdominal aortic aneurysm." *Cardiovascular and Interventional Radiology* 32 (2009): 535–8.

[18] Nault I, Miyazaki S, Forclaz A, Wright M, Jadidi A, Jais P, et al. "Drugs vs. ablation for the treatment of atrial fibrillation: the evidence supporting catheter ablation." *European Heart Journal* 31 (2010): 1046–54.

[19] Cox JL, Jaquiss RD, Schuessler RB, Boineau JP. "Modification of the maze procedure for atrial flutter and atrial fibrillation. II. Surgical technique of the maze III procedure." *Journal of Thoracic and Cardiovascular Surgery* 110 (1995): 485–95.

Klaudia Proniewska, Damian Dołęga-Dołęgowski,
Agnieszka Pręgowska, Piotr Walecki, and Dariusz Dudek

8 Holography as a progressive revolution in medicine

8.1 Introduction to holographic technology

The first studies about holographic technology can be found in the 1860s by British scientist John Henry Pepper. He developed a technique that we can now describe as a first example of the holographic type. Referred to as the "Pepper's Ghost," it was an illusion technique used in theaters. It relied on the use of two similar-sized rooms, light and a large plate of glass [1]. The audience watched the stage through a plate of glass set at the right angle (similarly to watching the road through cars' front window). A second, hidden, room was placed outside the audiences' field of view but in such a way that it was entirely visible through the plate of glass set on the stage. Properly decreased stage light and increased light in the "hidden" room caused the appearance of reflection on the plate of glass. Objects appearing on the glass were reflections of objects located in the "hidden" room. From the audiences' perspective, they looked like ghost objects standing on the stage (depending on the brightness of light, they've been more/less transparent). Such a technique of showing objects/information in the air/environment where they do not physically exist can be assumed as the basic definition of holography technology.

The first hologram was created in 1947 by Dennis Gabor, who was given the Nobel Prize in 1971 for this. And the first ideas for the use of this technology are noted in the films of the seventies. Lloyd Cross made the first moving hologram recordings, where subsequent frames with an ordinary moving film are applied to the holographic film. Nice-looking examples can be also found in *Star Wars: Episode IV*, where people communicate over very large distances using holographic audio-video connection displayed just in the air. So far, we are still far from making holograms just in the air without any additional displaying devices [2]. Moreover, holograms are used in video games such as *Command & Conquer: Red Alert 2, Halo Reach*, and *Crysis 2* [3].

Scientists are still working on obtaining the best quality/resolution of objects, but so far, the best realizations still rely on using glass plates, just like it was first shown by Pepper. Currently, most devices available on the market use a micro-projector (even 10× smaller than those seen in many home cinemas). The picture is displayed on specially developed prism glass (construction is very similar to typically used glasses) and it "stays" there. Depending on the manufacturer, we can find solutions that mainly use one or two glasses and a laser or projectors to display pictures. So far on the market, we can buy simple devices that just display information located statically in one place on the operator glasses, irrelevantly from the environment and objects located in the room. More advanced devices combine augmented reality (AR) and holography, where objects/pictures are displayed in a way that they cooperate with the real environment [4].

For example, a 3D designer develops an object on the computer and later displays it on the table in such a way that it pretends to be standing there [5]. One product that combines holography, AR, and portability is the Microsoft HoloLens [6]. This device includes double eye projectors for holography, multiple depth cameras (allows AR to map in a 3D environment and locate object to display in a way that it harmonizes with surroundings), microphone, and speaker for communication (for videoconference use). The entire process of generating objects, environment mapping, and other processing is done by a built-in microcomputer. Thanks to all of the above and a built-in battery, we now have access to powerful holographic glasses that can be used in almost every environment.

8.2 Augmented reality versus virtual reality

Virtual reality (VR) is a medium that can accomplish the embodiment, described by three features: immersion, presence, and interaction. The "immersed in the reality" experience created by computer technology was achieved by the maximum removal of sensations from reality and changing them with the observation from a virtual environment. Presence is a psychological phenomenon crucial to feel as in a virtual environment. Presence determines the level in which people being in a virtual environment react similarly as in the real world, revealing the same behavior and emotional and physiological responses. Therefore, presence is associated with a sense of involvement in the virtual world and being a part of it, which determines the place illusion and the plausibility illusion. These phenomena are related to the interaction, the ability of the computer to detect and respond to user actions in real time by responding appropriately to commands or customizing virtual character responses. Interacting with the virtual environment, even in an unreal way, is the key to a sense of presence.

Virtualization has been defined as "an activity in which man interprets the patterned sensual impression as a stretched object in an environment other than that in which it physically exists" [7]. In the virtual world, the participant is part of the environment, thanks to which head movements cause parallax of movement from the participant's point of view, and reactions related to focusing and tracking of objects are stimulated [8]. In VR, the experiment took place in a simulation that can be similar or completely different from the real world.

The main assumptions of VR are to simulate a place/location/situation for the user, who is not physically in there. For example, a person wearing a special VR helmet can picture himself riding a rollercoaster, whereas in reality, they are comfortably sitting in a chair in the office. The user is disconnected from their environment and only sees the image displayed by the VR helmet (Fig. 8.1). AR is the next technology developed after VR. The first sort of AR device was developed by Ivan Sutherland in 1968 [9], but the term "augmented reality" was first used in 1990 by Thomas Caudell and David Mizell from the Boeing company. In the beginning, the concept of AR is associated with a futuristic vision ever since. AR in some way is an extension of it. What is it? AR is an enhanced version of the physical world through the use of different stimuli such as audio or vision. Digital information is integrated with the user's environment in real-time. Today we are witnessing how it becomes a component of our almost everyday life [10]. AR is divided into three main categories, i.e., markerless AR (location-based, position-based, or GPS), projection-based AR (projects artificial light onto a real-world surface), and superimposition-based AR (it is possible to replace the original view of objects with AR objects).

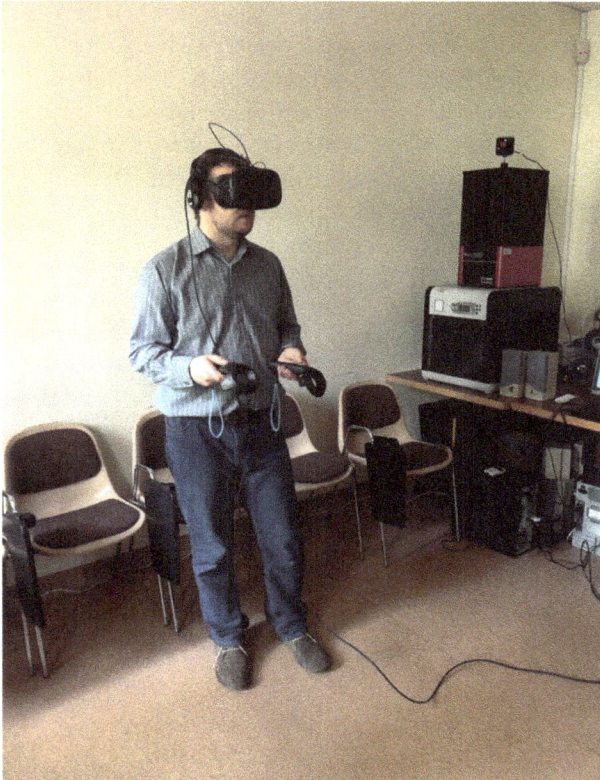

Fig. 8.1: HTC-Vive-Setup helmet and environment [own source].

AR is some ways a very similar technology; however, using special AR glasses or helmets, in the user still sees their real surrounding environment. It can be compared to using normal glasses. What is new in this technology? AR glasses display the image in a way that harmonizes with the environment. To summarize, VR moved the user into a completely different computer-generated world, such as Oculus Rift [11]. AR applies additional visual elements to the real world, such as Google Glass [12]. Two market-leading solutions are VIVE Pro from HTC [13] and the HoloLens [HoloLens] from Microsoft (Fig. 8.2). In contrast to VIVE Pro, HoloLens is independent and does not require manual controllers. The device is fully integrated with Microsoft Enterprise systems. Its interface is known to users using the Windows operating system on other computer platforms, which makes it easier for users to use it for the first time. The disadvantage of this solution is the fact that the commercial license for HoloLens has a much higher price than VIVE Pro (even taking into account the cost of a workstation computer) [14].

Microsoft HoloLens [6] is the world's first wireless holographic computer. It allows full control over holographic objects, enabling moving, changing their shape, and placing them in the mixed reality space. All equipment is housed in special glasses; no wires or additional devices are needed. For example, a person wearing AR glasses can see an object placed on his desk right in front of him, which physically is not there. Another feature is that AR allows to walk around the desk and watch such an object from different angles when the object is displayed in the glasses in a way that includes the distance of the user from his desk and also angle from which he looks it. In this way, the device can to create a new image each time the user moves, creating an illusion that an object exists in the users' environment without physically being there. A major benefit of AR, compared with VR, is that the user never loses his orientation in the environment where he is (Fig. 8.3).

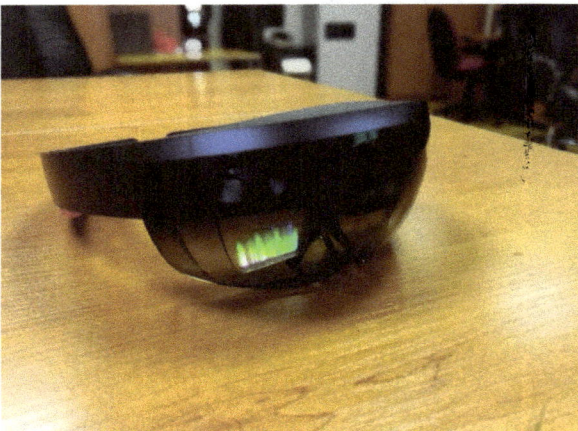

Fig. 8.2: Microsoft HoloLens—the world's first wireless holographic computer [own source].

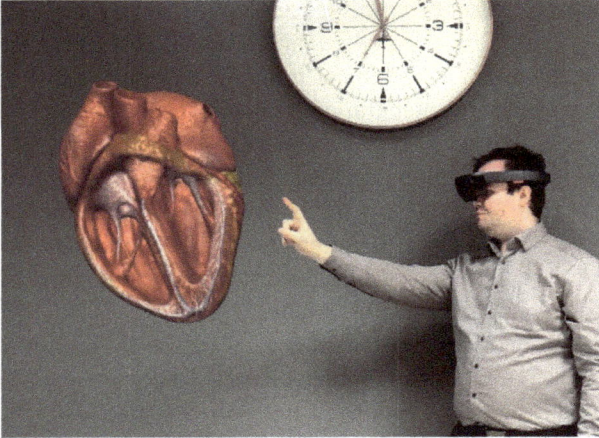

Fig. 8.3: Augmented reality glasses can display objects next to the person [own source].

8.3 AR, VR, and holograms for the medical industry

Suddenly, Holograms became a new buzz word when AR was a marketing mantra since 2016. Virtual and AR are immersive technologies that provide new and powerful ways for people to generate, use, and interact with digital information. Currently, every industry wants to see if you can use holograms to get specific benefits. Statista.com predicts that the size of the AR and VR market will increase from USD 27 billion (2018) to 209.2 billion (2022) [15].

Medicine is a discipline that a leader in testing innovative solutions, as well as their regular use in the diagnosis, therapy, and rehabilitation of patients. In this area, the most practical innovation is the application of mixed reality, or a combination of the real image and signals biological data with obtained data, e.g. during the diagnostic process using imaging techniques. AR takes an important role in many medical applications like laparoscopy, endoscopy, or catheterized intervention [16–19]. AR and VR research, once the domain of well-financed private institutions and organizations, is now democratized, and with the terminology.

8.4 Training and mode of action scenarios—medical VR/AR

Clinical staff members responsible for patient care meet with different scenarios in their daily work. Simulating complicated medical situations that require a combination of social, technical, and teamwork skills is a very interesting field in which you can apply AR, among others. These types of solutions can be implemented in the simulation of medical cases as a new form of medical education. New technologies give trainers full design freedom in terms of training scenarios reflecting the real working conditions of medical teams [20]. Currently, many academic centers want to test the possibility of using AR and VR in clinical training. Several important points must be taken into account in the preparation of medical applications in mixed reality:

a. There is a need for very high-resolution medical images, e.g., computed tomography (CT). Besides large 3D data sets (scans) may need to visualize. Can devices such as HoloLens meet these requirements? Videos provided on the Internet are a mix of high-quality images, but they seem to be marketing, in contrast to other, crueler (but more credible) possibilities.

b. Should optically transparent or digitally transparent devices be used? This again leads us to VR wearable devices HoloLens and Google Glass v/s, such as GearVR. At this point, it can compare two devices HoloLens and Google Glass (GearVR). Both have their pluses and minuses. Optically transparent naturally creates a less alienating experience, giving the user the opportunity to see the real world, we still do not know how high the fidelity is and these so-called light points— holographic density compared with the resolution captured images using digital AR solutions.

c. AR and VR have a problem with the delay, which can be less frustrating than the delay with optical visual equipment because the whole "world" will be synchronized with the person.

d. Currently, tests are being carried out on mobile devices, where the delay in updating was noticeable. It was a stress test for the mobile solution Mixed Reality; therefore, the optimization of models and resources is sought.

One of the advantages of the digital transparency of "mixed reality" compared with optical transparency is that the user can seamlessly "travel" between worlds. This is important in a training simulation, for example, if the training aims to take care of the victims in an epidemic or trauma. The simulation of mixed reality can include the following: mannequin placed on a green mat, which is then inserted into the VR world along with the chaos, which would be visible during the first aid medical situation. Such training simulations are most effective in VR. Digital transparency provides the ability to combine AR and VR to achieve a mixed reality. Another example is the administration of a drug to a patient (3D model of AR) imposed on a hospital bed and then a smooth tracking of the course of the drug into the blood vessels of patients and organs.

8.5 Teaching empathy through AR

During education, students reach the point where they have to understand how anatomy is made. Currently, students have a wide range of books, videos, lectures, and seminars from which they can learn. Besides that, during the practical exercises, under the supervision of experienced doctors, students get the possibility to develop their manual skills. Theoretical knowledge is not enough; students must have the well-developed spatial vision to imagine the course. To make it easier to understand and imagine it spatially, the holographic application was created. It was developed to work on Microsoft HoloLens devices. It displays data/application on user glasses in a way that it looks for a user like it would exist in the reality of our environment. The application allows to display 3D objects in a way that they can be rotated, zoom in/out, and also penetrate. Thanks to it, students learn basic pieces of information about the anatomy of pulp chambers and canals in a three-dimensional way.

To better understand holographic technology, it is good to review existing applications that use it. In this chapter, we will review a few different examples of medical applications developed especially for the holographic purpose and Microsoft HoloLens devices.

In 2016, Case Western Reserve University and Cleveland Clinic prepared a HoloAnatomy course (Fig. 8.4) [9]. McDuff and Hurter [21] proposed CardioLens, a mixed reality system using HoloLens, which is real-time, hands-free, and blood visualization from many people's lives. Ortiz-Catalan et al. [22] presented help to a phantom limb pain patient. They designed a new virtual environment in which the patient used his missing arm to use it to perform simple tasks such as lifting and moving small objects. A holographic prototype of the 3D digital anatomy atlas for neuroscience was created in 2016 by Holoxica Limited. Companies such as Medicalholocek.com (Switzerland), CAE Healthcare (USA), Pearson, SphereGen, Digital Pages (Brazil), and MedApp (Poland) use AR, and HoloLens glasses are for training purposes, including the visualization of human anatomy. DICOM Director (USA) enables communication and collaboration between different doctors and medical practitioners.

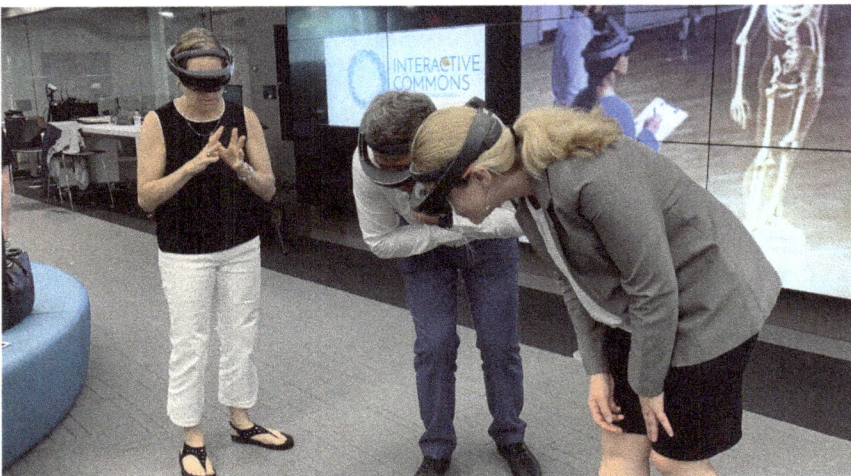

Fig. 8.4: Viewing objects in three dimensions helps to understand how they really appear. Interactive Commons, Case Western Reserve University, Cleveland Clinic, USA, 2019 [own source].

The application contains a very simple user interface and a very well made guide during the entire process of using the application. In the beginning, the user has to decide where he wants to have the generated model placed. To do that, the user only needs to look at pointing a dot at the right place and use a pointing gesture to confirm his selection. Everything else in the application can be done using voice commands. The application is made in a way that the user is guided through stories prepared by authors. This story/presentation shows a working way of using HoloLens with the human body. It has a few chapters where a guide talks about the human body with different 3D models displayed in holographic technology. Every chapter takes 1–2 min, and when the guide stops talking, the user is left with a holographic model to review/analyze it. To go to the next chapter, the user needs to say "next," and the application generates a new holographic model and talks about it [23]. The biggest benefit of prepared models is that they are done from many smaller objects. When the user approaches the human body, he will be able to see that bones, internal organs, or the circulatory system are separate models.

This is not the end; the user can penetrate the entire body by moving with glasses more into the model. Thanks to that feature, deep organs that are not visible at the beginning because they are covered by bigger organs can be seen. One of the chapters shows the brain with a tumor inside. This is something that for now could be only visible using magnetic resonance imaging (MRI) or computer tomography. In the holographic model, the user could see the entire brain tissue with around 50% of visibility and tumor, which was inside with 100% visibility. In this way, the user could see exactly how the tumor is placed and in which direction it is moving/attacking. It is important to mention at this time that the user can walk around every generated holographic model and watch it from every different direction/angle. For now, this application is used as an educational task. It is used for students of medicine to study the human body and learn it more practically, using holographic technology. Also, holography and AR technology will become the next-generation library.

8.6 Holography in the operating room

What can a combination of medicine and advanced information technology give? It gives breakthrough and revolution in caring for the sick and a completely new era in surgical techniques and imaging. Technologies that we once could see only in sci-fi movies become a reality today, for example, expanded or mixed reality using HoloLens goggles in the operating room. On March 2018, Professor Dariusz Dudek together with a team of doctors from the Jagiellonian University Medical College, Krakow, Poland, conducted the first in Europe treatment of atrial septal defect (ASD) using HoloLens technology in real-time. The treatment took place at the Second Clinical Department of Cardiology and Cardiovascular Interventions at the University Hospital in Krakow. On this day, at the same time, further consultations and treatments were held using innovative hologram-based imaging methods in Nowy Sacz, 100 km away. Thanks to the technology of the Kraków-based MedApp company on HoloLens, Prof. Dudek could connect with the center in Nowy Sącz in real-time for consultation and support on the treatment plan on an ongoing basis. The use of HoloLens and the ability to see a very accurate hologram of the heart revolutionize imaging in cardiology and surgical techniques (Fig. 8.5).

Would not it be great to perform a procedure on an organ (e.g., heart, liver, and teeth) and at the same time have access to an x-ray, CT, ultrasound, or another image, e.g., augmented visualization? Data visualization techniques using AR give us the opportunity to access a dedicated organ. Thus, using AR, it is possible to visually evaluate the external and internal structures of the object (Fig. 8.6). The introduction of this new technique requires the use of properly prepared equipment and dedicated software. The basic equipment is the glasses, which impose a virtual image selected from images on the image seen in real, which were used, for example, in the diagnosis process [24].

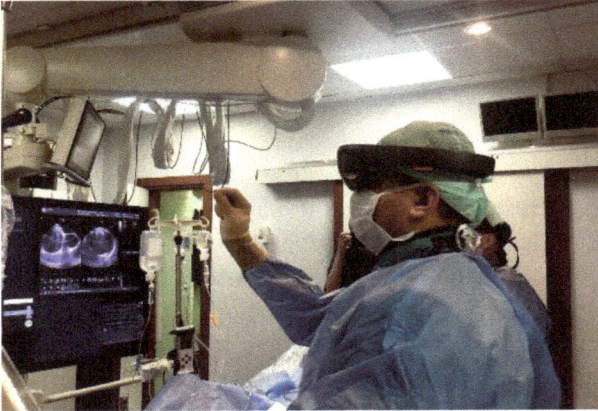

Fig. 8.5: Case study—atrial septal defect (ASD). Operator: Professor Dariusz Dudek, Jagiellonian University Medical College, Krakow, 2018 [own source].

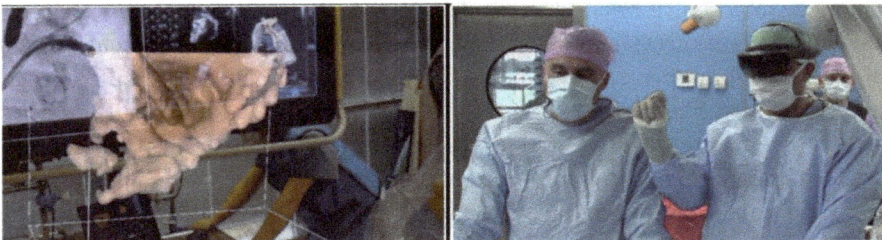

Fig. 8.6: Case study—left atrial appendage hologram HoloLens assistance. New Frontiers in Interventional Cardiology Workshops, Krakow, 2018 [own source].

Thanks to the introduction of the latest technologies in the education process, we indicate the path of development in medicine and shape in the students of medicine the desire to enjoy the benefits of new technologies.

In turn, in July 2017, neuroradiology's Wendell Gibby performed an operation on the lumbar region spine using Microsoft HoloLens. To precisely locate the drive that caused back pain, MRI images and CT were loaded to the OpenSight software and then visualized in the 3D image of the spine. After applying HoloLens, the doctor could see the patient's spine superimposed (displayed) like a film on his body. HoloLens tracked the location, to which the doctor watched and navigated the anatomy with more accuracy. Also, Beth Israel Deaconess Medical Center, Visual 3D Medical Science and Technology Development CO. LLC (China) and AP-HP (France) carry out surgical procedures using HoloLens.

The groundbreaking AR/mixed reality technology of the HoloLens reality that allows the visualization of anatomical and pathological structures of patient's organ reflects a modern approach to "tailor-made" patient care, that is, the maximum individualization tailored to a given patient [25, 26].

8.7 Medical holographic applications—our team examples

8.7.1 A wireless heart rate monitor integrated with HoloLens

The HoloLens device made by Microsoft [6] changes the way how we can perceive information, for example, doctor documentation working space. The basic idea of a holographic assistant for a doctor was described in our previous paper [27]. The proposed solution removes almost everything from the doctor's desk. No cables, monitors, or even a mouse or keyboard is needed. Thanks to holographic technology, we receive multiple screens around the doctor's desk. A number of them can be selected in a way that doctors like: one huge screen or maybe four smaller screens with different pieces of information on each of them. Doctors decide what exactly they need at the moment: RTG photo, treatment history, or maybe a schedule of visits to plan the next appointment, everything available just in front of a doctor. High importance information is displayed in front of the doctor to remind about some patient pieces of information, for example, the dangerous reaction for anesthetics, heart problems, or HIV and AIDS sickness when doctors should engage with high caution. The biggest advantage of this way of working is that all of the pieces of information are visible only for the doctor and no one else. The device is secured with a built-in monitor checking if the device was taken off from the doctor's head, which results in blocking access to the application. Another example of holography can be found in Poland, where application and hardware to allow user/doctor monitor patient pulse was developed. The entire idea of the system was to show that thanks to holography and wireless technology, a doctor can watch a patient, read the documentation on the patient's examination and all the time be able to see his pulse value (Fig. 8.7) [27].

During the patient's visit, a wireless heart rate sensor is placed on their finger. The microcomputer connected to that sensor collects data and sends the result to the HoloLens' application started on HoloLens. The entire communication is done over a WiFi connection. The application on HoloLens displays "on-air" actual heart rate value, and information (name) of the patient is exanimated (information is taken from an existing database). The application does not contain any other interface that could limit the field of view for a doctor. This is another big feature where doctors receive additional information without losing their eyeshot.

The entire idea of this solution is aimed to show a way that every patient can be monitored in real-time by a doctor wearing only a holographic device (Fig. 8.8).

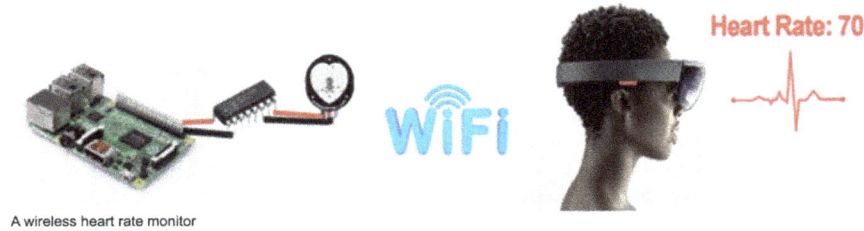

A wireless heart rate monitor

Fig. 8.7: A wireless heart rate monitor integrated with HoloLens [29] [own source].

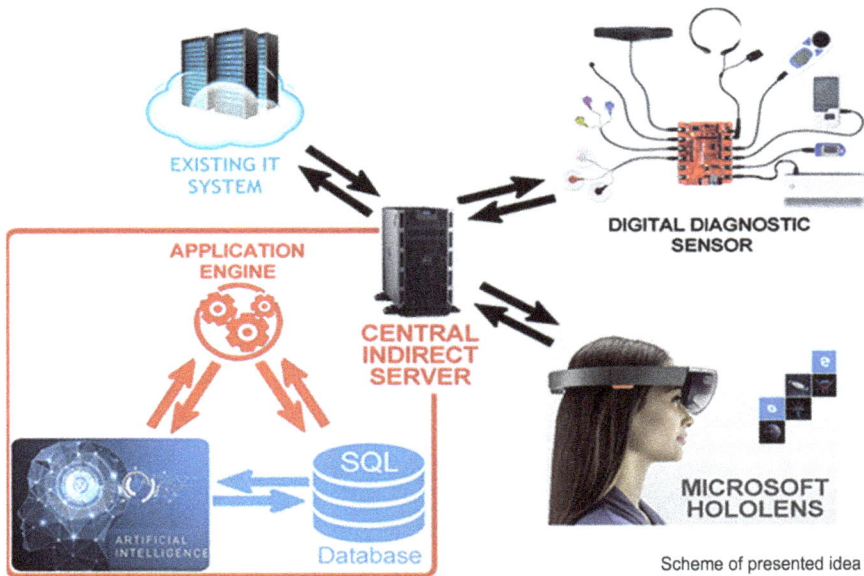

Scheme of presented idea

Fig. 8.8: Scheme of digital diagnostic sensor monitor integrated with HoloLens [29] [own source].

A doctor can examine all types of different patient parameters, blood tests, or other results of the examination by having them in front of him. The digitalization of medical documentation is already ongoing. Papers disappear from doctors' desks. The General Data Protection Regulations restricts a way how medical clinics should manage patient documentation in a way that holography is starting to become the best solution for this. The Microsoft HoloLens device restricts what is visible and by who it can be accessed. A doctor can have in front of him many different restricted documents that only he can see.

8.7.2 Holography in stomatology

We tested the feasibility of using HoloLens during carrying out tooth morphology (Fig. 8.9). All people using HoloLens were amazed by the technology and 3D models that they could experience from different angles. Everyone agreed that this is something that could simplify and help during their studies when they had to learn root canals paths.

The created application was done in a few steps. First, 3D models of root canals with different paths where the canals can go were created. It had to include the situation when canals connect, separate, or even change their direction. All of that was done according to Vertucci's classification. The entire work was done using Autodesk Maya, the software typically used to create 3D models for games and animations. When models where done, they were exported to Unity software. It is an application used to create video games and AR software for different devices and systems. A huge benefit of this application is that it also allows creating AR applications

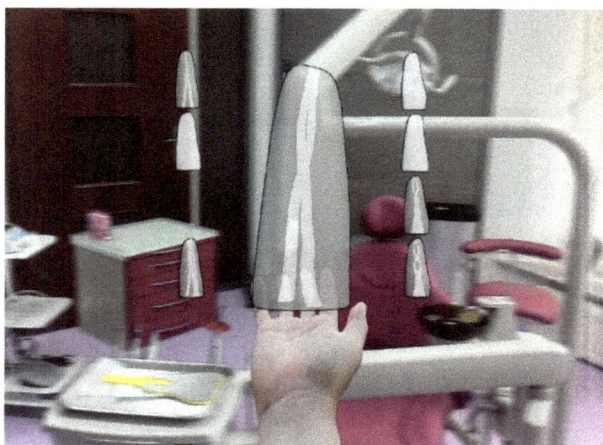

Fig. 8.9: Experimental holographic setup. 3D models of root with different paths of how canals go own [own source].

for the Microsoft HoloLens device. Thanks to it, models created in Maya could be imported to this project. Next, it was required to create separate scripts
- to place models in the exact position in the user-visible area (anchoring models to our environment so they stay in one place),
- to animate action for clicked/selected object (root) in a way that it moved to the middle of the screen and change its size to bigger and start rotating,
- to animate actions for returning the root to its place and mark it as already used/selected, and
- to inform the main management which root was selected so they would know where to put it back.

After testing the application in the Unity emulator, the final step was to export the ready project to Microsoft Visual Studio. This development software is responsible for the final compilation process in a way that application could be installed on the Microsoft HoloLens device.

8.8 Future perspectives: visualization of anatomical structures

The new generation of equipment for displaying holographic objects gives the opportunity to visualize anatomical structures in the form of an interactive three-dimensional image based on scans from classic medical imaging. The visualization of medical data and the ability to view in space, as well as the possibility of cutting anatomical/pathological structures, are reference points for doctors. This is a new innovation in the field of interpretation of medical data. The solution for the visualization of the patient's internal organs, both anatomical and pathological structures, using the latest devices is a reflection of modern technologies used in medicine. The proposed technology leads to the implementation of individualized diagnostics of the latest achievements in data visualization techniques in three dimensions. What will the future bring? We will see. One thing is for sure, holography is on its way to revolutionizing medicine.

8.9 References

[1] http://scihi.org/john-henry-pepper-peppers-ghost/ (accessed October 11, 2019).
[2] Screen grab from *Star Wars: Episode IV—A New Hope*.
[3] Johnston SF. "Channeling Dreams." In *Holograms: A Cultural History*. Oxford University Press, 2015.
[4] http://holocenter.org/what-is-holography (accessed October 11, 2019).
[5] https://interactive-commons.webflow.io (accessed October 11, 2019).
[6] https://www.microsoft.com/en-us/hololens (accessed October 11, 2019).
[7] Ellis SR. "Nature and origin of virtual environments: a bibliographic essay." *Computing Systems in Engineering* 2 (1991): 321–47.

[8] Sanchez-Vives MV, Slater M. "From presence to consciousness through virtual reality." *Nature Reviews Neuroscience* 6, no. 4 (2005): 332–9.

[9] Sutherland IE. "A head-mounted three-dimensional display." In *Proceedings of the Fall Joint Computer Conference*, pp. 757–764. Washington, DC: Thompson Books, 1968.

[10] Bach B, Sicat R, Beyer J, Cordeil M, Pfister H. "The hologram in my hand: how effective is interactive exploration of 3D visualizations in immersive tangible augmented reality?" *IEEE Transactions on Visualization and Computer Graphics* 24 (2018):457–67.

[11] https://www.oculus.com/ (accessed October 11, 2019).

[12] https://www.google.com/glass/start/ (accessed October 11, 2019).

[13] https://x.company/glass/ (accessed October 11, 2019).

[14] Orgon D. "HoloLens and ViVE Pro: virtual reality headsets." *Journal of the Medical Library Association* 107, no. 1 (2019): 118–21.

[15] https://www.statista.com/statistics/591181/global-augmented-virtual-reality-market-size/ (accessed October 11, 2019).

[16] Azuma R, Baillot Y, Behringer R, Feiner S, Julier S, MacIntyre B. "Recent advances in augmented reality." *IEEE Computer Graphics and Applications* 21 (2001): 34–47.

[17] Silva R, Oliveira JC, Giraldi GA. *Introduction to Augmented Reality*. National Laboratory for Scientific Computation, Av Getulio Vargas, 2003.

[18] Sielhorst T, Feuerstein M, Navab N. "Advanced medical displays: a literature review of augmented reality." *Journal of Display Technology* 4 (2008): 451–67.

[19] Carmigniani J, Furht B, Anisetti M, Ceravolo P, Damiani E, Ivkovic M. "Augmented reality technologies, systems and applications." *Multimedia Tools and Applications* 51 (2011): 341–77.

[20] https://realvision.ae/blog/2016/04/mixed-reality-ar-vr-holograms-medical/ (accessed October 11, 2019).

[21] McDuff D, Hurter Ch. *CardioLens: Remote Physiological Monitoring in a Mixed Reality Environment*. ACM SIGGRAPH 2017 Emerging Technologies, 2017.

[22] Ortiz-Catalan M, Sander N, Kristoffersen MB, Hakansson B, Branemark R. "Treatment of phantom limb pain (PLP) based on augmented reality and gaming controlled by myoelectric pattern recognition: a case study of a chronic PLP patient." *Frontiers in Neuroscience* 25 (2014): 8–24.

[23] EDUCASE Review. *Mixed Reality: A Revolutionary Breakthrough in Teaching and Learning*. https://case.edu/research/sites/case.edu.research/files/2018-08/Mixed%20Reality_%20A%20Revolutionary%20Breakthrough%20in%20Teaching%20and%20Learning%20_%20EDUCAUSE.pdf (accessed October 11, 2019).

[24] Tepper OM, Rudy HL, Lefkowitz A, Weimer KA, Marks SM, Stern CS, Garfein ES. "Mixed reality with HoloLens: where virtual reality meets augmented reality in the operating room." *Plastic and Reconstructive Surgery* 140, no. 5 (2018): 1066–70.

[25] Mitsuno D, Ueda K, Hirota Y, Ogino M. "Effective application of mixed reality device HoloLens: simple manual alignment of surgical field and holograms." *Plastic and Reconstructive Surgery* 143, no. 2 (2019): 647–51.

[26] Moosburner S, Remde C, Tang P, Queisner M, Haep N, Pratschke J, Sauer IM. "Real world usability analysis of two augmented reality headsets in visceral surgery." *Artificial Organs* (2018) [Epub ahead of print].

[27] Proniewska K, Dołęga-Dołęgowski D, Dudek D. "A holographic doctors' assistant on the example of a wireless heart rate monitor." *Bio-Algorithms and Med-Systems* 14, no. 2 (2018): UNSP 20180007.

Joanna Szaleniec and Ryszard Tadeusiewicz

9 Robotic surgery in otolaryngology

9.1 Introduction

This chapter is about surgical robots and their applications in otolaryngology. Surgical robots are different from the robots widely used in the industrial applications. Industrial robots are programmed for performing some technological manipulations and production operations, which after programming are being done automatically and repetitively for many fabricated products. Such scheme of robot use is illustrated in Fig. 9.1.

However, such scheme was not proper for the use of the robots in surgery. In industrial applications, the task is easier. Every fabricated element is identical; therefore, the sequence of operations performed by robot for every fabricated element can be the same. The sequence of actions performed by robot can be programmed once and executed many times. In surgery, the situation is different. Every human body is different, and every lesion is different. It means that for every operation, robot should be programmed separately. It is very inconvenient. Therefore, during the surgical use, robot is controlled by the surgeon. The structure of such control system is presented in Fig. 9.2. The work of the surgeon is easier and more comfortable than during traditional surgery because instead of standing at the operating table, they can sit comfortably by a special control console. Moreover, the computer that controls the movements of surgical instruments inserted into the patient's body through the robot's arms can perform very precise movements related to the operation. The ratio between the surgeon's hand movement on the manipulator in the robot control console and the movement of the surgical tool controlled inside the patient's body can be 1:10, which allows obtaining unattainable precision in the cutting and sewing of the operated tissues. The computer can also completely eliminate these surgeon movements, which can have a detrimental effect on the outcome of the operation, for example, hand tremor or accidental excessive movement that may lead to damage to adjacent organs. The surgeon can see the surgical field and every movement of surgical instruments because the robot has TV cameras and special illuminators on one of the arms inserted into the patient body, and the console is equipped with a vision system presenting images from the inside of the patient's body stereoscopically and (if necessary) enlarged (up to 30 times). One of the illuminators is a laser-emitting monochromatic light that allows you to notice the course of blood vessels inside the operated organ.

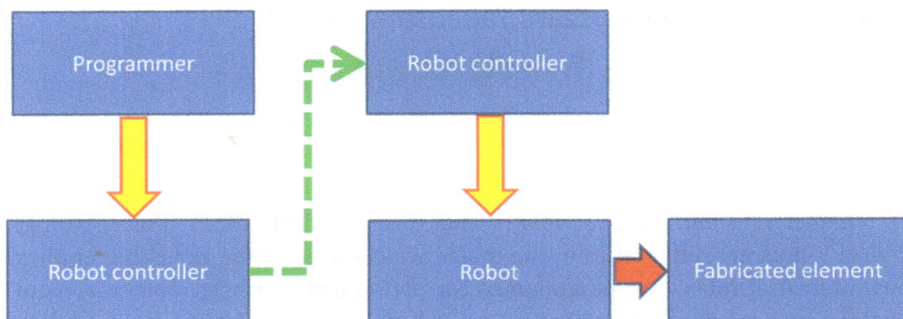

Fig. 9.1: Scheme of typical industrial robot use. Source: own elaboration.

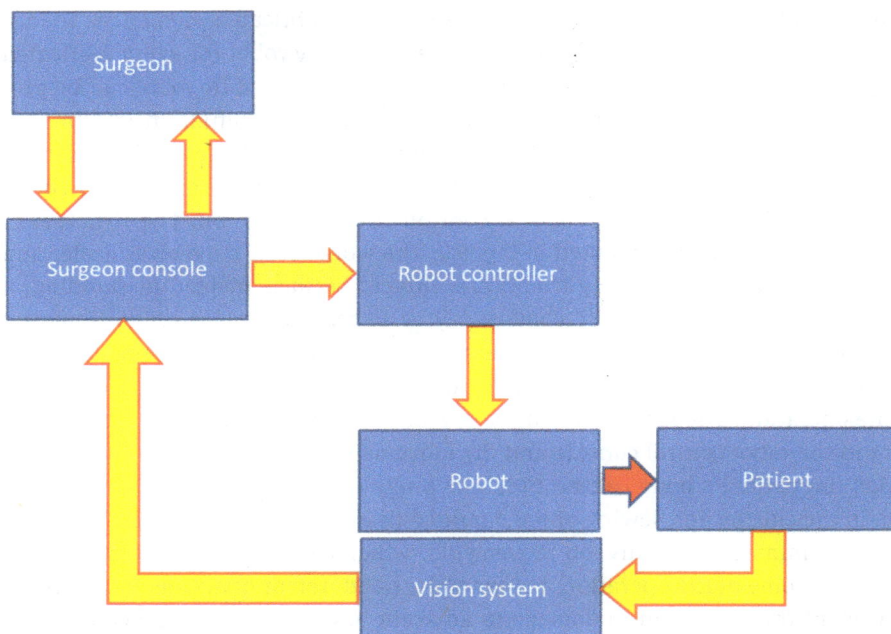

Fig. 9.2: Scheme of typical surgical robot. Source: own elaboration.

Finally, it can be concluded that the surgical robot does not present such a level of automation of the activities performed that is achievable using industrial robots. It is actually an intelligent manipulator, not a robot in the full sense of the word. However, the use of this tool is very purposeful because it guarantees better results from the patient's point of view (the surgical procedure is less invasive and can be more precisely carried out) and for the surgeon (more comfortable work).

9.2 General remarks

The first use of robot during a surgical operation probably occurred on March 12, 1984, at the UBC Hospital in Vancouver. The robot (named *Arthrobot*) was used in an orthopedic surgical procedure [1]. After this success, over 60 arthroscopic surgical procedures were performed in the same hospital in the following year. In 1985, an industrial robot, the Unimation Puma 200, was used to navigate a needle for a brain biopsy under CT guidance during a neurological procedure [2]. A robotic system for commercial use was first developed in 1995. The history of robotic surgery, the description of the structure and functions of surgical robots, and the detailed descriptions of the methodology of robotic surgery in urological applications were presented in book [3]. The removal of a cancerous prostate has been a popular robot-assisted treatment, but there are numerous other applications. In general, robot-assisted surgery can be used for heart surgery, thoracic, gastrointestinal, gynecological, orthopedic surgery, and many others. Examples of the use of robotic surgery systems in heart surgery are described by Mayer et al. [4]. Robots are used for three heart surgery types: atrial septal defect repair, mitral valve repair, and coronary artery bypass. The robotic heart surgery is part of more general area of robotic thoracic surgery, described by Melfi et al. [5].

Also, a very broad area of robotic surgery applications is connected with gastrointestinal surgery [6] as well the robotic surgery in gynecology [7]. However, these interventions will not be considered in this chapter of the book.

The first surgical robots were invented also for telesurgery, with an intention to operate astronauts in the orbit or soldiers wounded on remote battlefields [8]. In fact, remote robotic surgery has actually never been performed in space for astronauts. The number of robot teleoperations in military applications is not known because of military secrecy. Therefore, the first (and famous) official teleoperation using surgical robot was conducted on September 7, 2001. This operation was conducted through the Atlantic Ocean and was named Operation Lindbergh after Charles Lindbergh's pioneering transatlantic flight. The surgeon (Jacques Marescaux) was in New York and the patient was in Strasbourg. Computer Motion's *Zeus* robot was used, and the performed teleoperation was a cholecystectomy. The scheme of this pioneering operation is presented in Fig. 9.3.

9.3 Robotic surgery in head and neck—advantages and disadvantages

The main problem, considered in this chapter, is the application of surgical robots in head and neck surgery. The general overview of this problem was presented by Garg et al. [9]. The most widely used robotic system in otolaryngology is the da Vinci Surgical Robot (Intuitive Surgical Inc., Sunnyvale, CA, USA), and the majority of the surgical procedures are performed via the oral cavity (transoral robotic surgery [TORS]).

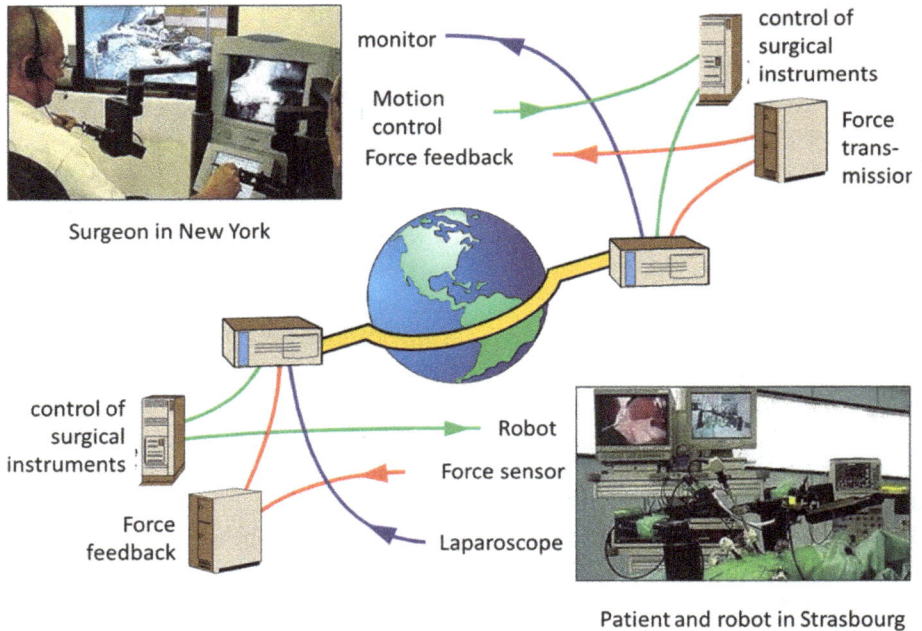

Surgeon in New York

Patient and robot in Strasbourg

Fig. 9.3: Remote surgery with the robot use. Source: own elaboration.

The system has been approved by the Food and Drug Administration for head and neck surgery in 2009.

The da Vinci system includes three components [3, 10]:
(1) a surgical cart with a robotic manipulator and three arms (one for a camera and two for other instruments; the instruments have several degrees of freedom to mimic the movements of the human wrist) (Fig. 9.4)
(2) a vision cart that provides visualization (two cameras in one endoscope)
(3) a surgeon's console with a three-dimensional stereoscopic viewer (Fig. 9.5)

Robot-assisted surgery can be particularly useful in the head and neck region for several reasons [11]:
(1) Robotic surgery allows for minimally invasive procedures. In open approaches, the incision needs to be wide enough to ensure direct visualization of the surgical field. Endoscopic approaches (including those applied for robotic surgery) require only minimal "keyhole" incisions to introduce the camera and the surgical devices. For intranasal and intraoral procedures, the endoscopes are introduced through natural openings and may not require any additional tissue damage to provide adequate visualization. The reduction of the surgical incision size is extremely important on the head and neck, where the scars are usually

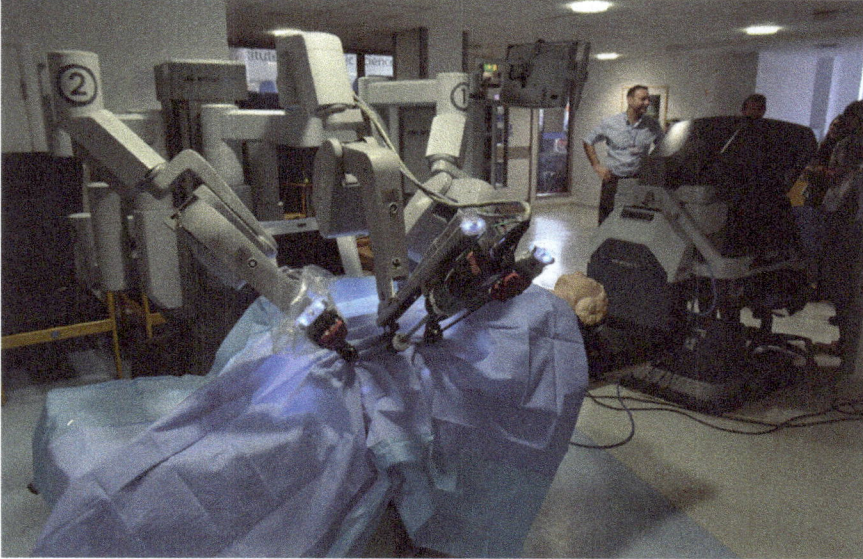

Fig. 9.4: da Vinci surgical cart. Source: https://upload.wikimedia.org/wikipedia/commons/2/23/ Cmglee_Cambridge_Science_Festival_2015_da_Vinci.jpg. This file is licensed under the Creative Commons Attribution-Share Alike 3.0 Unported license.

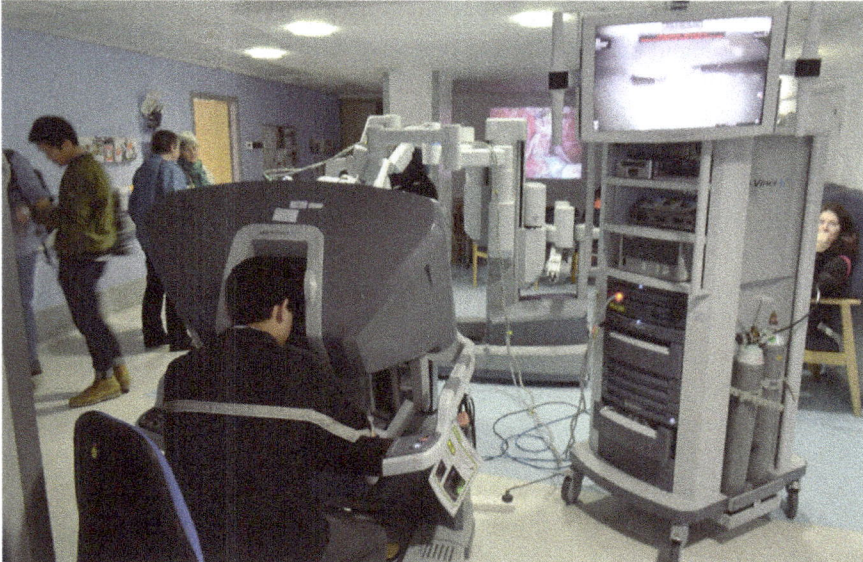

Fig. 9.5: Surgeon console in the da Vinci robot system https://upload.wikimedia.org/wikipedia/ commons/6/68/Cmglee_Cambridge_Science_Festival_2015_da_Vinci_console.jpg. This file is licensed under the Creative Commons Attribution-Share Alike 3.0 Unported license.

readily visible. Open surgical procedures, especially on the face, frequently cause scarring that may be hardly acceptable for the patient.

(2) The anatomy of the head and neck is very complex, and many vital structures are located very close to one another. In classic approaches (without angled endoscopes and instruments), it is sometimes difficult or even impossible to avoid damage to the nerves or blood vessels or other structures that "stand in the way." It is not uncommon that gaining access to the pathology can cause more damage than the procedure itself [12]. This problem can be (literally) circumvented if robotic surgery is applied. One of the most important advantages of TORS is the fact that even extensive procedures can be completed without the necessity to perform mandibulotomy (incision of the mandible) that is often necessary in open procedures. Minimally invasive procedures ensure better functional results and improved quality of life.

(3) The head and neck surgeon frequently has to operate in confined spaces, and microsurgery constitutes an important part of everyday otolaryngological practice. Three-dimensional visualization with sufficient magnification provided by the robotic system helps the surgeon to precisely maneuver the instruments in microscale. Moreover, the system eliminates the tremor of the surgeon's hand. As the instruments are not directly handheld, large movements of the surgeon's hand can be translated into much smaller and more precise movements in the surgical field ("motion scaling") [12].

(4) Surgical approaches to the head and neck are frequently uncomfortable for the surgeon. For example, during endonasal or transoral procedures, the surgeon often needs to bend over the lying patient and remain in a forced position to introduce the instruments and endoscopes at the required angles. The hands holding the endoscope and other instruments are not supported. Therefore, prolonged operations may cause fatigue and reduce the quality of the surgeon's performance. In robotic surgery, the remote workstation allows for a comfortable and ergonomic position (seated position with supported forearms and head).

(5) Currently, endoscopic surgery is the gold standard for many procedures in otolaryngology. Endoscopic surgery has several drawbacks compared with robotic surgery. In endoscopic procedures, one hand has to hold the endoscope, which leaves only one hand free to manipulate the tissues. Besides, the endoscopic visualization lacks the third dimension that is frequently crucial for adequate assessment of the surgical field. The surgical robots provide both bimanual manipulation and three-dimensional visualization.

(6) Many surgical procedures in the head and neck are optimally performed with surgical lasers. The robotic systems allow for better maneuverability of the laser tip and improve the visualization of the area of resection. Traditionally, the laser has to be used in the line of sight. The robotic arms allow for working at different angles or even "around corners" [13].

However, the application of the da Vinci system has also several disadvantages:
(1) One of the most important factors limiting the access to surgical robots in many countries is the high price of their installation and maintenance. Therefore, the cost-effectiveness of these devices is frequently questioned. Besides, the equipment needs a lot of space in the operating room—a requirement that may not be fulfilled in many hospitals.
(2) Robotic surgery requires special training of the surgeon and assistant personnel. Some surgeons are unwilling to learn a new skill, which requires time and effort. However, the robotic system allows the trainee to be supervised by an experienced colleague at another console or to use a virtual training environment. The learning curve for surgeons already trained in transoral surgery was shown to be short [14].
(3) The setup of the system and the exposure of the surgical field are time consuming and prolong the time of operation, especially if the personnel is still learning how to operate the system [15].
(4) The surgeon has to rely only on the visual feedback without tactic or haptic sensation. After classic training, the surgeon is accustomed to use the sense of touch to examine the tissues or adjust the force applied with the instruments. To operate a robotic system, one needs to change these habits.
(5) The access to the surgical field provided by the robotic system can turn out to be suboptimal in certain patients. Patients with mandibular deformities or trismus may require conversion from an transoral approach to open procedures [16].
(6) The robot is too bulky to be used for some endonasal or otologic procedures [17].

Some of the limitations of the da Vinci robot were addressed in the next robotic system (FLEX Robotic System) designed and manufactured by Medrobotics Inc. (Raynham, MA). It provides high flexibility and maneuverability, and its smaller size makes it easier to fit in most operative rooms. The access of both the camera and the instruments to the surgical site is nonlinear. The surgeon can easily maneuver around anatomical structures, which makes the system very well suited for transoral procedures. The FLEX system can also provide some haptic feedback [18].

9.4 Applications of the da Vinci system for head and neck surgery

The da Vinci system was first applied in the head and neck region by Haus in animal models in 2003 [19]. Its first application in a human patient was a transoral excision of a vallecular cyst performed by McLeod and Melder in 2005 [20]. This pioneer operation was also preceded by studies in porcine and cadaveric models because the da Vinci system was originally designed for much wider surgical fields (abdomen and thorax) and adjusting its setup for airway surgery proved to be challenging [21].

In the same year, Hockstein, Nolan, O'Malley and Woo tested the de da Vinci robot on an airway mannequin to define the optimal method of exposure for microlaryngeal surgery. Traditionally, endolaryngeal procedures are performed via a laryngoscope. Its narrow closed tube does not provide enough space to introduce the large robotic arms and ensure an adequate range of their movements. The authors concluded that the best access was provided by a mouth gag with cheek retractors, a tongue blade and a 30-degree endoscope [21]. Later, the same authors tested the setup described above on a cadaver and proved that the exposure was sufficient to perform several endolaryngeal and pharyngeal surgical procedures. They also observed that the wristed instruments (with tips that can bend at required angles) allowed for manipulations that would be much more difficult or even impossible with traditional rigid instruments introduced via a laryngoscope. This feature of the da Vinci robot was found very promising because it could facilitate endoscopic management of lesions that would otherwise require open procedures [22]. Further experiments were conducted by Weinstein, O'Malley, and Hockstein in canine models [23, 24].

9.5 Transoral robotic operations

The most common use of medical robots in head and neck surgery is connected with TORS. In 2006, the preclinical studies were followed by transoral robotic excisions of T1-T2 tongue base malignant tumors in three human patients. It was possible to perform complete *en bloc* resections, whereas the transoral laser surgery usually requires piecemeal or cutting through tumor resection. There were no complications and adverse events. The authors claim that robotic excision was less technically challenging than endoscopic laser procedures. They also observed that TORS offered better options for hemostasis than endoscopic surgery [25].

In 2007, the robotic technology for TORS was successfully coupled with CO_2 laser technology [26].

In subsequent years, the scope of robotic surgery expanded even further. TORS was used for supraglottic partial laryngectomy [27], radical tonsillectomy for previously untreated invasive squamous cell carcinoma of the tonsillar region [28], and oropharyngeal carcinoma, including advanced T4 tumors [29, 30] in much larger groups of patients. Disease control, survival, and safety were similar to standard treatments, and the number of patients that required a gastrostomy after oropharyngeal cancer excision was even lower than for standard nonsurgical therapies.

TORS was shown to have the benefit of shorter hospital stay and fewer postoperative complications when compared with open approaches [31]. A recent analysis of over 2,000 TORS patients compared with over 6,000 nonrobotic surgery patients operated for early stage oropharyngeal cancer in the United States showed that the advantages of robotic surgery were lower likelihood of postsurgical positive margins and subsequent need for adjuvant chemoradiotherapy [32].

More and more challenging transoral robotic procedures are still being developed. Recently, even a total transoral laryngectomy was shown to be feasible; however, it seems to be reasonable primarily in these rare cases when concurrent neck dissection is not necessary [33–36].

9.6 The FLEX system

The application of the FLEX robotic system for transoral surgery was first tested on human cadavers in 2012 [37]. The endolarynx was easily visualized without laryngeal suspension. Subsequently, the robot's efficacy was shown in several endolaryngeal, laryngopharyngeal, and oropharyngeal procedures [38]. In 2014, FLEX received the CE approval and was used for the first surgeries in human patients [39]. The robot was used for transoral surgery for oropharyngeal tumors [40]. The use of the considered robot for first 40 operations was described by Mattheis et al. [41]. This robot was also used in the United States [42]. It was evaluated as easy to setup, precise, and safe.

9.7 Conclusion

The examples of successful applications of two different types (da Vinci and FLEX) of surgical robots for head and neck surgery show that robotic surgery can be used, and should be used, in otolaryngology. Currently, the limit is the very high price of a surgical robot, which means that only very rich hospitals can afford this type of technical support for doctors. However, one can hope that the numerous advantages of surgery using robots (described in the Introduction) will lead to a wider use of this method of performing surgical operations, and also in the field of laryngology.

9.8 References

[1] Lechky O. "World's first surgical robot in B.C." *The Medical Post* 21, no. 23 (1985): 3.
[2] Kwoh YS, Hou J, Jonckheere EA, Hayati S. "A robot with improved absolute positioning accuracy for CT guided stereotactic brain surgery." *IEEE Transactions on Bio-Medical Engineering* 35, no. 2 (1998): 153–60. doi:10.1109/10.1354. PMID 3280462.
[3] Dobrowolski Z, Tadeusiewicz R, Glazar B, Dobrowolski W. *Robotic Urology* [In Polish: Robotyka urologiczna]. Krakow: Lettra-Graphic, 2014 (ISBN: 78-83-89937-70-4).
[4] Mayer H, Gomez F, Wierstra D, Nagy I, Knoll A, Schmidhuber J. "A system for robotic heart surgery that learns to tie knots using recurrent neural networks". *Advanced Robotics* 22, nos. 13–14 (2008): 1521–1537. doi:10.1163/156855308X360604.
[5] Melfi FM, Menconi GF, Mariani AM. "Early experience with robotic technology for thoracoscopic surgery." *European Journal on Cardio-Thoracic Surgery* 21 (2002): 864–8.

[6] Talamini MA, Chapman S, Horgan S, Melvin WS. "A prospective analysis of 211 robotic-assisted surgical procedures." *Surgical Endoscopy* 17, no. 10 (2003): 1521–4. doi:10.1007/s00464-002-8853-3. PMID 12915974.

[7] Liu H, Lawrie TA, Lu D, Song H, Wang L, Shi G. "Robot-assisted surgery in gynecology." *Cochrane Database of Systematic Reviews* 12, no. 12 (2014): CD 011422. doi:10.1002/14651858. CD011422. PMID 25493418.

[8] Choi PJ, Rod J, Oskouian RJ, Tubbs RSh. "Telesurgery: past, present, and future." *Cureus* 10, no. 5 (2018): e2716, doi: 10.7759/cureus.2716, PMCID: PMC6067812.

[9] Garg A, Dwivedi RC, Sayed S, et al. "Robotic surgery in head and neck cancer: a review." *Oral Oncology* 46, no. 8 (2010): 571–6.

[10] McLeod IK, Melder PC. "Da Vinci robot-assisted excision of a vallecular cyst: a case report." *Ear, Nose and Throat Journal* 84, no. 3 (2005): 170–2.

[11] Oliveira CM, Nguyen HT, Ferraz AR, Watters K, Rosman B, Rahbar R. "Robotic surgery in otolaryngology and head and neck surgery: a review." *Minimally Invasive Surgery* 2012 (2012): 286563. doi: 10.1155/2012/286563. Epub 2012 Apr 10.

[12] Mack MJ. "Minimally invasive and robotic surgery." *JAMA* 285, no. 5 (2001): 568–72.

[13] Hockstein NG, Nolan JP, O'Malley BW Jr., Woo YJ. "Robotic microlaryngeal surgery: a technical feasibility study using the da Vinci Surgical Robot and an airway mannequin." *Laryngoscope* 115, no. 5 (2005): 780–5.

[14] Lawson G, Matar N, Remacle M, Jamart J, Bachy V. "Transoral robotic surgery for the management of head and neck tumors: learning curve." *European Archives of Oto-Rhino-Laryngology* 268, no. 12 (2011): 1795–801.

[15] McLeod IK, Melder PC. "da Vinci robot-assisted excision of a vallecular cyst: a case report." *Ear, Nose and Throat Journal* 84, no. 3, (2005): 170–2.

[16] Weinstein GS, O'Malley BW Jr., Cohen MA, Quon H. "Transoral robotic surgery for advanced oropharyngeal carcinoma." *Archives of Otolaryngology—Head and Neck Surgery* 136, no. 11 (2010): 1079–85.

[17] Garg A, Dwivedi RC, Sayed S, et al. "Robotic surgery in head and neck cancer: a review." *Oral Oncology* 46, no. 8 (2010): 571–6.

[18] Poon H, Li C, Gao W, Ren H, Lim CM. "Evolution of robotic systems for transoral head and neck surgery." *Oral Oncology* 87 (2018 Dec): 82–8. doi:10.1016/j.oraloncology.2018.10.020. Epub 2018 Oct 25.

[19] Haus BM, Kambham N, Le D, Moll FM, Gourin C, Terris DJ. "Surgical robotic applications in otolaryngology." *Laryngoscope* 113, no. 7 (2003 Jul): 1139–44.

[20] McLeod IK, Melder PC. "Da Vinci robot-assisted excision of a vallecular cyst: a case report." *Ear, Nose and Throat Journal* 84, no. 3 (2005): 170–2.

[21] McLeod IK, Mair EA, Melder PC. "Potential applications of the da Vinci minimally invasive surgical robotic system in otolaryngology." *Ear, Nose and Throat Journal* 84, no. 8 (2005 Aug): 483–7.

[22] Hockstein NG, Nolan JP, O'Malley BW Jr., Woo YJ. "Robot-assisted pharyngeal and laryngeal microsurgery: results of robotic cadaver dissections." *Laryngoscope* 115, no. 6 (2005): 1003–8.

[23] Weinstein GS, O'Malley BW Jr., Hockstein NG. "Transoral robotic surgery: supraglottic laryngectomy in a canine model." *Laryngoscope* 115 (2005): 1315–9.

[24] O'Malley BW Jr., Weinstein GS, Hockstein NG. "Transoral robotic surgery (TORS): glottic microsurgery in a canine model." *Journal of Voice* 20, no. 2 (2006): 263–8.

[25] O'Malley BW Jr., Weinstein GS, Snyder W, Hockstein NG. "Transoral robotic surgery (TORS) for base of tongue neoplasms." *Laryngoscope* 116, no. 8 (2006): 1465–72.

[26] Solares CA, Strome M. "Transoral robot-assisted CO_2 laser supraglottic laryngectomy: experimental and clinical data." *Laryngoscope* 117, no. 5 (2007): 817–20.

[27] Weinstein GS, O'Malley BW Jr., Snyder W, Hockstein NG. "Transoral robotic surgery: supraglottic partial laryngectomy." *Annals of Otology, Rhinology and Laryngology* 116, no. 1 (2007): 19–23.

[28] Weinstein GS, O'Malley BW Jr., Snyder W, Sherman E, Quon H. "Transoral robotic surgery: radical tonsillectomy." *Archives of Otolaryngology—Head and Neck Surgery* 133, no. 12 (2007): 1220–6.

[29] Moore EJ, Olsen KD, Kasperbauer JL. "Transoral robotic surgery for oropharyngeal squamous cell carcinoma: a prospective study of feasibility and functional outcomes." *Laryngoscope* 119, no. 11 (2009): 2156–64.

[30] Weinstein GS, O'Malley BW Jr., Cohen MA, Quon H. "Transoral robotic surgery for advanced oropharyngeal carcinoma." *Archives of Otolaryngology—Head and Neck Surgery* 136, no. 11 (2010): 1079–85.

[31] Weinstein GS, O'Malley BW Jr., Desai SC, Quon H. "Transoral robotic surgery: does the ends justify the means?" *Current Opinion in Otolaryngology and Head and Neck Surgery* 17, no. 2 (2009): 126–31.

[32] Li H, Torabi SJ, Park HS, Yarbrough WG, Mehra S, Choi R, Judson BL. "Clinical value of transoral robotic surgery: nationwide results from the first 5 years of adoption." *Laryngoscope* 21 (2018 Dec). doi: 10.1002/lary.27740. [Epub ahead of print].

[33] Lawson G, Mendelsohn AH, Van Der Vorst S, Bachy V, Remacle M. "Transoral robotic surgery total laryngectomy." *Laryngoscope* 123, no. 1 (2013): 193–6. doi:10.1002/lary.23287.

[34] Dowthwaite S, Nichols AC, Yoo J, Smith RV, Dhaliwal S, Basmaji J. "Transoral robotic total laryngectomy: report of 3 cases." *Head Neck* 35, no. 11 (2013): E338–42. doi:10.1002/hed.23226.

[35] Smith RV, Schiff BA, Sarta C, Hans S, Brasnu D. "Transoral robotic total laryngectomy." *Laryngoscope* 123, no. 3 (2013): 678–82. doi:10.1002/lary.23842.

[36] Krishnan G, Krishnan S. "Transoral robotic surgery total laryngectomy: evaluation of functional and survival outcomes in a retrospective case series at a single institution." *ORL Journal for Oto-rhino-laryngology and Its Related Specialties* 79, no. 4 (2017): 191–201. doi:10.1159/000464138.

[37] Rivera-Serrano CM, Johnson P, Zubiate B, Kuenzler R, Choset H, Zenati M, Tully S, Duvvuri U. "A transoral highly flexible robot: novel technology and application." *Laryngoscope* 122, no. 5 (2012 May): 1067–71. doi:10.1002/lary.23237. Epub 2012 Mar 23.

[38] Johnson PJ, Rivera-Serrano CM, Castro M, Kuenzler R, Choset H, Tully S. "Demonstration of transoral surgery in cadaveric specimens with the medrobotics flex system." *Laryngoscope* 123 (2013): 1168–72.

[39] Remacle M, Prasad VMN, Lawson G, Plisson L, Bachy V, Van Der Vorst S. "Transoral robotic surgery (TORS) with the Medrobotics Flex System: first surgical application on humans." *European Archives of Oto-Rhino-Laryngology* 272 (2015): 1451–5.

[40] Mandapathil M, Duvvuri U, Güldner C, Teymoortash A, Lawson G, Werner JA. "Transoral surgery for oropharyngeal tumors using the Medrobotics® Flex® System—a case report." *International Journal of Surgery Case Reports* 10 (2015): 173–5.

[41] Mattheis S, Hasskamp P, Holtmann L, Schäfer C, Geisthoff U, Dominas N. "Flex Robotic System in transoral robotic surgery: the first 40 patients." *Head Neck* 39 (2017): 471–5.

[42] Persky MJ, Issa M, Bonfili JR, Goldenberg D, Duvvuri U. "Transoral surgery using the Flex Robotic System: initial experience in the United States." *Head Neck* (2018). doi:10.1002/hed.25375.

Jan Witowski, Mateusz Sitkowski, Mateusz K. Hołda,
Michał Pędziwiatr and Marek Piotrowski

10 Hospital management

10.1 Hybrid rooms

The rapid development of minimally invasive techniques, as well as imaging systems with the possibility of image fusion from various devices, and the possibilities of integrating and managing medical devices have made the traditional operating room concept find its complement in the form we call *hybrid room*. It is therefore an operating room where treatments are performed in the form of a hybrid (combination): minimally invasive procedures (e.g., coronary vessel diagnostics—coronary angiography and angioplasty treatment) with the possibility of performing full surgical procedures (including cardiosurgical procedures). The concept of a hybrid room is quite ambiguous; there are no detailed requirements or guidelines regarding its equipment. It is assumed, however, that such a room must be equipped with a device enabling blood vessel imaging such as an angiograph (one- or two-plane). Quite often, the concept of hybrid type rooms is also used when there is a large diagnostic device (e.g., MRI or CT scanner) in the operating room. These and other devices (such as endoscopic imaging systems, intraoperative microscopes, and ultrasound scanners) should be able to interact and communicate with one another, for example, by means of data exchange or by overlapping (merging) images. The combination of many techniques significantly improves diagnostic quality, increases the precision and effectiveness of treatments, and makes treatments shorter and less invasive. The large accumulation of equipment, however, means that rooms of this type need special methods of equipment planning and device placement, or even the way of moving and communicating between the staff of various specialties (surgeons, anesthesiologists, consultants of selected fields, and nursing and technical staff). A hybrid room is therefore a specific place where ergonomics and regulations from many fields of medical engineering should be taken into account (e.g., radiological protection, medical gases, ionizing radiation, electromagnetic field, complicated laminar airflow supply systems, and other climatic conditions). Among other devices, in addition to the aforementioned equipment, the hybrid room usually includes the following: a surgical lamp (usually a dual head with the ability to record and transmit audio and video signals); a set of (anesthesiological and surgical) power columns equipped with medical gas outlets, power sockets, fasteners, apparatus for general anesthesia, and vital signs monitoring; resuscitation and anesthetic equipment (defibrillator, suction pump, respirator, and set of infusion pumps); electrosurgery system (available in many forms, e.g., as a classic electrosurgical knife, jet surgery knife, plasma knife, ultrasonic knife, or using other technology); cardiology equipment (counterpulsation controller, turbine hemopump, extracorporeal circulation pump, autotransfusion device, and blood coagulation monitor); and a set of surgical instruments and other small equipment (e.g., infusion fluid heaters, patient heaters, functional furniture, tool tables, and containers). For the efficient and safe management of such a technology-saturated zone, the operating room management systems discussed below are being used more and more often. It should be anticipated that the concept of hybrid rooms, which for many years has usually belonged to cardiac disciplines, will quickly evolve toward other specialties that use advanced intraoperative imaging techniques. Hybrid rooms closely cooperate with or are even created as an integral part of the integrated room systems described below. Because of the accumulation of equipment and installations for the correct and safe operation of the hybrid room, it is necessary to properly organize its work allowing free movement of both equipment and medical personnel without restrictions in access to the patient. To optimize the costs, however, it is advisable that the hybrid rooms can also function as standard operating rooms, which can be achieved, for example, by appropriate selection of equipment allowing its easy rotation. In the future, one can expect the development of hybrid rooms technology in the direction of large-area rooms where even several treatment and diagnostic devices will be grouped, e.g., a tomograph, an angiography (or a hybrid of both), or various versions of MRI devices. It will be a natural development in the direction that became the determinant of this technology at the beginning of its implementation, that is, especially the constant increasing of the diagnostic and treatment potential within the operating room, which significantly increases the effectiveness of the procedure, reduces the number of additional procedures that should be performed outside the operating room, and accelerates the ability of the operating team for quick intervention.

10.2 Integrated rooms

The increasing amount of medical equipment within operating rooms means that integration systems are becoming an increasingly common standard especially in the operating blocks of several or a dozen or so rooms. The operating room integration system in the basic version usually has such functions as control from a touch All-in-One computer installed on the power column or another place indicated by the user, graphical and text control interface, video module for preview, control, recording and playback of recorded images from several connected sources, an audio module for capturing, recording of sound reproduction, and a module for controlling medical devices operating in the operating room (e.g., lamps, columns, electrosurgical systems, tables, etc.), which should be a modular structure element allowing expansion for subsequently introduced devices. The integration system should also have or be ready to be expanded with the control of infrastructure elements such as a medical gas module and electric power lines within operating rooms or devices securing climate parameters required by medical equipment suppliers and ensuring adequate work comfort for users and a patient. The application controlling the system should have an intuitive graphical control interface that provides control of all system functions, the function of assigning an operated patient to a specific surgical operator, including the possibility of individual system configuration depending on the needs and selected functions. The system control can be done on touch and conventional devices. Typically, it is implemented by a set of devices in the following configuration: a touch screen panel installed in an operating room on an additional arm on the power column or in another place convenient to control with a resolution in min full HD class, built-in high-capacity hard disk, integrated graphics module, min 8GB RAM memory, a set of USB, RJ-45, HDMI, DPx1, line-out or other types of signal inputs, and other controls like the keyboard and mouse connected via a USB port with protection rating of min IP65.

In the case of operating blocks consisting of a larger number of rooms, each of them is an integrated unit but has communication with others through technical cabinets (the so-called rack). Thus, it is possible to redirect the captured data, images, and films to any of the monitors inside the room, and to other rooms, conference rooms, doctors' offices, etc. In addition to elements permanently connected with the infrastructure (like surgical lamps or power columns), devices that can be integrated within the management system include, among others, X-ray machines, surgical microscopes, anesthetic and life-monitoring devices, navigational systems, and surgical robots. In addition to device control and the ability to transmit audio-video data, these systems may have or cooperate with external digital systems for managing medical data that are also used for recording, archiving, and processing of images and video sequences from recorded surgical procedures. Events are recorded on digital media, e.g., CDs, DVDs, memory cards, and other devices connected via USB ports. These images can then be viewed on external computers and dedicated media players or directly in the system. The system allows saving photos and video images, and it also allows adding descriptions, analyses, and interpretations with the possibility of editing and later access. Systems integrating the management of medical devices within the operating rooms also evolve toward other areas, e.g., as management systems for endoscopy laboratories. In this case, in addition to the standard functions of medical instrument management, the tracking process is important, which is the system for tracking endoscopes, which reduces the risk of infections and is a tool for decision-making support in the event of occurrence of such an event (determining who and when was in contact the instrument, who and in what moment carried out individual processes). This type of information can be in fact generated automatically, thanks to an access system that recognizes equipment and service at every stage (washing, drying, storage, and dispensing of equipment). In the case of large amount of equipment, the introduction of an automated control system minimizes the effect of human errors and constitutes a significant contribution to the documentation of the entire surgical process, increasing the probability of its safe conduct.

10.3 Surgical robotics

More and more commonly used surgical robots, despite the differences in their design, specific to each manufacturer, have several common elements, which can include the following:
- operator console
- robotic instrument arms with auxiliary elements, e.g., endoscopic camera
- high-resolution video system
- a set of reusable surgical instruments (forceps, blades, handles, etc.)

The robotic instrument arms of the robotic system can be integrated into the main unit as well as a set of interchangeable and independent arms in which surgical instruments or endoscopic devices are placed. In the case of a modular system, the operator determines how many arms will be active during the current treatment.

The operator console should provide vibration reduction to minimize natural hand shake and accidental movements, and to scale instrument motion proportional to the operator's movements. It should take into account the individual parameters of the operator (body structure, movement mechanics, and ergonomic position during the procedure), faithfully reproduce the tactile sensations, recognize and eliminate accidental movements, and control various system elements such as instruments or camera. Depending on the design of the robot, the control levers mimic the actual movements of the operator's hands (i.e., movement of the operator's hand to the right causes the instrument to move to the right, and movement of the operator's hand to the left causes the instrument to move to the left), enabling the surgeon to control the instruments and the endoscopic camera inside the patient's body, or offer a solution in which the console handles transmit the movement of the operator's hand to the movement of the active instrument in a manner corresponding to the natural movements of laparoscopic instruments during the surgery and react to the touch and pressure of the instrument tip on the tissue even outside the operator's field of view so as to minimize the risk of damage (perforation) during the procedure. Simultaneous control of visualization and surgical instruments can be aided by eye tracking functions that are used to adjust the field of view (zoom in, zoom out), and by moving the endoscope, it is possible to assign instruments to the most appropriate robot arms.

The design of the console should make it possible to obtain a comfortable, ergonomic position during the procedure performed by adjusting the console position to the operator's body structure. The operator, sitting comfortably behind the console, should be able to issue instructions for devices connected to the robot's individual arms using drivers on the console. In addition to a typical desktop that contains the control levers and control buttons for adjusting the operating parameters, power buttons, or emergency switch, an important control element is the footswitch panel. It is placed at the base of the surgical console, acting as an interface enabling the performance of various surgical operations (camera control, coupling of main controllers, arm switching, and control of electrosurgical devices). There is also a solution in which the footswitch panel located on the basis of a surgical console allows configuring a set of foot controllers controlling various functions of devices in the operating set and includes a foot switch controlling the system's safety system enabling stopping (freezing the position of instruments) at any moment of the treatment to improve the position of the operator's hand or in the event of the need to perform other activities related to the safety of the procedure. The control panel, e.g., in the form of a touch screen, should enable a selection of various system functions (including camera/endoscope settings, advanced video parameter adjustments, display preferences, audio settings, account management, record management, and preferences regarding system control parameters). In systems with independent modules, in which each arm is equipped with a movable base allowing any arm location, each base includes its own touch panel. It controls the arm setting and the emergency switch, and it also has a communication interface with the central system unit and base-stabilizing system in the place of its setting and interlocking. The advanced system function adjustments, including account management, operator login to the system, and preferences regarding system control parameters, can be controlled using the keyboard on the operator console.

The system should allow changing the patient's position during a procedure performed using a standard operating table. This also applies to laparoscopic procedures—its construction should ensure that in an emergency the instruments will be easily removable from the patient's body and the patient should be able to safely change position (without the need to disassemble the robot arms operating the patient). The instruments used should be reusable instruments with the possibility of sterilization (there are also reusable solutions with a limited number of applications after which the instrument cannot be used, which is explained by the quality of treatments and prevention of nosocomial infections). In each of these solutions, however, it should be possible to sterilize in line with commonly available sterilization technique standards. This also affects the economy of the system used, especially in the long-term profitability and amortization analysis in relation to operating costs.

The control of the instrument arms and the camera arm can be done by synchronizing several elements such as adjusting joints, integrated instrument arms, camera arm, and electrically assisted or relying on the cooperation of several robotic arms located independently around the operating table, each of which can operate a surgical instrument or a camera depending on the configuration chosen by the operator. To increase the freedom of the system, the arms may have telescopic elements for adjusting the height and the range of the arm. Joints are then used to set the arms on a surgical platform to establish a central point, or a solution is also possible in which the arm joints enable the desired setting of the instrument or the instrument relative to the camera, and the button on each arm allows determining the "central" point for each selected instrument.

All control functions are supported by an electric drive—it allows docking and/or changing the position of the surgical platform. In the case of an integrated system, the electric drive interface includes a steering column, a throttle valve, a throttle opening switch, and displacement switches, while a solution, where each arm of the surgical platform is equipped with a movable platform enabling free positioning of the arms relative to the operated patient depending on the type of procedure performed. The electric drive of each platform enables the precise positioning of the arm and stabilization/locking it at the place of installation.

The robotic system works with a high-quality video system to process and transmit video information during the procedure, the elements of which are as follows: system core, light source, stereoscopic camera head, camera control system (connected to the camera via a single cable, controlling acquisition and processing of camera image), endoscope, video system trolley—central set for processing and displaying images, touch screen (for setting system parameters and viewing the image of the operating field), and fixtures for CO_2 tank. In addition, it should be possible for the system to be integrated with existing video systems adopted and used by the hospital for visualization during surgeries. It is also important to equip the system with a simulator for learning and to assess the operator's manual efficiency.

Apart from robots of a general surgery nature, robots dedicated to specific medical specialties are also becoming more and more common applications. One of the examples can be a neurosurgical robot designed for surgery within the head and spine areas. They allow performing procedures such as neuronavigation, biopsy, SEEG, DBS, or neuroendoscopic procedures. The robotic arm supported by a mobile trolley, which is also used to integrate the control and computing platform, is coordinated by means of hydraulic cylinders, providing several degrees of freedom of movement in space, including linear motion. The basic elements of the robot for this purpose are as follows:

- articulated arm for rigid attachment of the work handle and controlling neurosurgical instruments in accordance with the operation plan
- computer system for surgical planning, navigation, and stereotaxy, enabling the import of CT and MRI images, as well as enabling the design and saving of patient folders containing planned trajectories, markers, and other operational areas
- mechanical probe to locate anatomical structures during neuronavigation and a set of instrument adapters to adapt surgical instruments of various shapes and sizes
- optical distance sensor for the noncontact location of anatomical structures, for automatic registration without markers and hands-free navigation;
- calibration tools for manual recording of X-ray images in 2D
- mechanical holder for precise mechanical steering of the neurosurgical endoscope during chamber procedures and adapter for adapting a specific endoscope model, positioned by the robotic arm in accordance with the preoperative plan

- numerous modules of specialized software used, among others, for manually registering the patient's position using skin markers, matching automatic registration without markers; for merging multiple sets of patient data, enabling the manual setting of several multimodal images (CT or MRI) using anatomical landmarks; for surgical planning in functional neurosurgery, enabling the setting of images the patient; for endoscopic neurosurgery, enabling specific surgical planning, neuronavigation, and robotic manipulation of an endoscope, which enables determination of safety zones for each trajectory and advanced modes of manipulation of the endoscope using automatic movements.

An example of another specialized surgical robot is a system designed for ENT. This type of system not only must work in a straight line but also must apply to flexible surgery, i.e., in such specialties as head and neck surgery (through transoral approach) and in colorectal surgery (through transanal access), as well as in gynecology, thoracic surgery, and percutaneous general surgery. Systems can also be used for treatments in subsequent surgical specialties, including urological procedures. Treatments in all of the mentioned specialties are performed by the same robotic system, and only disposable tips and instruments are adapted to the requirements of a given specialty.

Systems of this type are developed in areas inaccessible in a straight line, like large intestine or airways, and thanks to the construction with a flexible arm allowing both visualization and conducting surgical procedures in the anatomical areas invisible and inaccessible in a straight line through the natural openings of the body, access is possible to areas with complex access routes in a virtually noninvasive manner.

Systems of this type have or cooperate with optical navigation systems, which plan an examination based on diagnostic tests (e.g., CT). They allow, among others, for planning the procedure through the outline with an indicator of the anatomical structures of the head with the sound effect signaling the correctness of the process and other activities such as calibration of any number of surgical instruments, application of multiple-use markers, automatic recording of surgical procedures with a built-in camera, an interface allowing easy adjustment of the procedure to the needs of the user in terms of instrument and treatment profile, the possibility of spatial 3D rotation and reconstruction, automatic zoom of operated structures, and image processing by adjusting parameters such as brightness, contrast, zoom, rotation, mirroring, and even a view from the perspective of the introduced instrument within structures. The specific type of navigation cooperating with robotic systems is intraoperative radio navigation. It is a gamma ray detector on the boom with an arm that can be controlled (e.g., by means of an electromagnetic system), and its operation is based on a scintillation lens made of CsI (Na) and photomultiplier sensitive to changes in position. Imaging of isotope-saturated areas takes place in real time on monitors, which means that the removed change is immediately visible on the

screens without having to rescan the area. A wide spectrum of markers should cooperate with the device, which allows the detection of many areas (e.g., sentinel lymph
node, head and neck tumors, thyroid and parathyroid tumors, breast tumors, prostate
tumors, endocrinology tumors, or other deep tumors). The auxiliary elements of such
a system are lasers with positioning function and external gamma radiation probes
for open and laparoscopic surgery displaying the results of measurements directly on
the surgical radionavigation screen.

In the case of endoscopic procedures, robotic systems can be in the form of
automatic optics positioners. Robotic optics positioner is a system in the form of
an arm, fastened to the table rail in any place with the possibility of remote control
without the help of an assistant. Communication with the device can be done by
voice activation, and additional control is carried out using a sterilizable joystick.
The system should be able to change the position of the "trocar point" at any time
during the procedure and provide a large range of motion that allows a full 360°
view with the inclination of the endoscope as much as possible. This type of system
can be mounted to the operating table or have a mobile stand for transporting and
storing the arm.

Surgical robotics also develops outside of the traditional operating rooms, an
example of which is a cyberknife. It is a device located in radiotherapy laboratories,
dedicated to noninvasive radiosurgery with the possibility of irradiation from many
directions using a robotic arm with many degrees of freedom. The apparatus enables
irradiation with the OMSCMRT method (image-monitored stereotactic and cybernetic
microradiotherapy), where the radiation source are photons with the energy of 6 MeV.
Thanks to its construction, the system allows irradiation in any plane without the
need to move the patient, keeping the position of the therapeutic table unchanged. In
this way, it is possible to apply the therapy with multiple isocenters and one isocenter,
and the total error of determining the location of the tumor is reduced to a tenth of
a millimeter. Because of the size and weight of the device and its components, the
apparatus must have an anticollision system preventing the patient from touching
the moving parts of the system. Movements of the robotic arm are closely correlated
with the patient position control system using a minimum of two images taken at different angles to obtain spatial information. The position control system is integrated
with the therapeutic device with respect to the possibility of automatically changing the position of the patient or changing the position of the apparatus during the
irradiation procedure in case of finding a change in the position of the tumor. Therefore, it is possible to take pictures during the irradiation procedure without having
to interrupt it, and the control of the location of tumors does not require the use of
markers and eliminates artifacts of tumor movements caused by respiratory movements. This in turn requires another integration within the entire system, namely,
with the therapeutic table. The integration enables the correction of the location of
the patient relative to the radiation source, determined based on the performed position control, which allows the patient to be automatically positioned in the correct

position to conduct therapy and automatic table movements performed without the operator entering the therapeutic room. This is also ensured by the extensive movement of the board—vertical, transversal, longitudinal, and revolutions—around the long axis of the table, around the axis perpendicular to the long axis of the table and its twisting. In addition to the typical mechanics and automation of movements of all components, an integral part of the robotic radiotherapy system must be a treatment planning system. It should provide the following elements: fusion of images from various imaging devices (CT/NMR/PET in the DICOM version 3.0 and DICOM RT format); planning 3D dose distributions, including nonuniform density; contouring of anatomical structures and areas for treatment; calculation and optimization of dose distribution; viewing and editing of treatment plans (dose schedules, DVH); the possibility of contouring on cross, frontal, sagittal, and oblique sections; the possibility of calculating dose distributions; and various optimization methods, including one in which the objective function includes the optimization of the total number of monitor units.

Other areas of interest for the development of robotics are the areas where the preparation of cytotoxic drugs takes place. Because they are classified as dangerous, carcinogenic, teratogenic, and mutagenic drugs, their preparation takes place in the premises of hospital pharmacies, which require special preparation and control. Efforts to effectively reduce the exposure of people working on their production led to the emergence of production and use of a system referred to as a robot for the production of cytostatics. The system prepares substances using a robotic arm, and the individual stages of preparation are controlled by sensors and elements of the video system. The system consists of the main unit, in which preparation, production, storage, dispensing of the finished drug, and waste securing take place, as well as a computer control system together with a set of devices for air treatment (pipes, ventilation, fans, HEPA H14 class filters, roof panels, etc.). The robotic part is equipped with a gripper cooperating with a dispensing device suitable for syringes of various sizes, a bar code reader for incoming products and an automatic, rotating magazine. Because of the specifics of the products, the system should have a number of monitoring and control elements, e.g., a syringe location system, a multistage filtration system, a UVC lamp system to prevent the growth of bacteria, and temperature, pressure, and airflow monitoring devices. The system is able to perform chemotherapeutic drug preparations through the implementation of many automated procedures, e.g.,

- collecting from the magazine for all materials needed for production;
- positioning the material in dedicated containers;
- material recognition and verification;
- automatic dosing, aspiration of the drug or its excess, introduction into the final packaging;
- automatic collection of waste, including closing, sealing, and storage;
- positioning and dispensing of preparations.

Irrespective of the robotization of the production procedures themselves, the system should have software for managing both semifinished products and ready-made drugs, cooperating with the pharmacy management system as a whole.

10.4 Patient verification systems

As the elements supporting the operation of this type of devices as well as the entire oncological therapy process, patient verification systems can be applied to control and identify the patient, for example, using a hand blood vessel scanner. The system can use, as a reference image, elements of the patient's body contours imported in the DICOM RT format as well as an image of the patient's surface collected by the system during the previous positioning or during positioning on a computer tomograph. Its construction is based on a three-dimensional imaging system in the visible light of the patient's body surface for the purpose of positioning and verification of the patient's position in real time using a set of high-sensitivity cameras observing the patient's body along its entire length and allows
- graphic displaying (visualization) of mismatch areas with an indication of the direction of the suggested correction of the body position of the patient;
- defining several areas of observation and verification in the field of camera system imaging;
- functions of automatic sending of an alarm signal in the case of motion detection outside the defined tolerance range;
- detection of patient's respiratory movements based on observation of the patient's body surface in a noninvasive and noncontact manner, without the need to use any additional accessories such as markers, belts, etc.,
- the ability to generate automatic reports at every stage of planning and performing therapy.

In addition to checking and verifying the patient, it is possible to use the system for the automatic control of parameters of radiotherapy treatments. A specialized dosimetry system offers for this purpose the possibility of automatic control of radiotherapy treatment parameters in real time, registering information about each segment of the applied beam. Constant and automatic control includes the shape, size, and position of the beam as well as the radiation dose. All these parameters are tracked with very high spatial resolution and sensitivity and compared with the treatment plan recorded in the DICOM RT system.

After automatically importing the patient's treatment plan, the parameters of the expected beam for each segment are automatically calculated, and after it is completed, the system is ready to analyze the course of the irradiation process. During the procedure, the analysis results are displayed in the form of tables and graphs on the control monitor.

If the dose received by the patient, i.e., its shape, size, or location in space in any segment, exceeds the margin set by the therapist, the system immediately alerts it through a sound signal, which allows the therapist to stop the irradiation immediately. All these activities are fully automatic and do not require any interference from the therapist. The system indicates an area incompatible with the planned one, i.e., whether the problem related to the shape of the field of irradiation, its size, or the dose rate that was delivered to the patient. This information can also be very helpful for the accelerator service. In the case of failures, they indicate the place where the problem occurred, which can greatly speed up the removal of the fault.

The verification of the delivered dose to the patient is the final stage of quality control of patients irradiation with external beams. In addition to controlling the patient's position, aimed at ensuring geometric compliance of the therapy with the treatment plan, it is one of the most important steps in quality control.

The advantages of this type of systems are as follows:

a. They enable the verification of the compliance of exposures with the treatment plan in real time (additionally, there is a possibility of interrupting irradiation in case of incorrect realization of the exposure).

b. They are characterized by very high sensitivity in detecting discrepancies between the actual state and the planned state (the ionization chamber is a very sensitive and reliable radiation detector).

c. They are characterized by a wide range of use of the device (it can be used to carry out quality control tests of therapeutic devices to verify treatment plans before its start, etc.).

10.5 Management systems for surgical instruments

At least the partial robotization of procedures is also taking place in other areas of hospitals. An example may be the management systems for surgical instruments and the circulation of other material subject to sterilization within a central sterilizer and operating block. Its basic functional features usually include the following:

– Observation of current sterilizers, washer—disinfectors, other devices by direct connection with device controllers in real time

– Monitoring the work of washers—disinfectors, autoclaves in a continuous manner—displaying the device status, monitoring errors and information in standby mode and during operation

– Registration of disinfector and autoclave washer processes and archiving of these parameters

– Registration of all washer errors—disinfectors and autoclaves

– Documentation of receipt of material for the Central Sterilization Department, external release documentation using barcode scanners

- Documentation of the instrument treatment process within the Central Sterilization Department with the assignment of activities to the personnel performing it physically using barcode scanners
- Storage of all information about individual instruments, kits, packaging materials, personnel, devices, and processes carried out on them in a single database on the server
- Possibility of automatic searching of batches by the system after defining parameters such as date and time, machine name, program name, batch status, and batch number
- Identification with access codes to the appropriate levels of competence for the staff operating the system together with the possibility of logging into the system using a barcode scanner
- Identification of packages based on the serial number assigned
- Possibility of documentation of instrument repair processes within the Central Sterilization Department and external services, documentation of issuing instruments for repair and their return, performed using barcode scanners
- Possibility of interactive packaging of the set by the user, using the on-screen packing list, verification of each type of an instrument, modification of the quantitative composition including the actual number of instruments
- The possibility of graphical presentation and storage of process flow charts carried out in washers, disinfectors, and sterilizers
- Possibility to create cost statements divided into groups depending on the size of the package
- Printing the table of contents of the set on laser printers
- Enabling tracking of the path of a set or instrument within the Central Sterilization Unit and to the patient and back
- Ensure the elimination of issuing of nonsterilized items to the recipient, and issue to the wrong recipient
- Possibility to modify and enter new data on instruments, kits, packaging, and recipients, regardless of activities performed on other computer stations
- Creating own queries/rules in the system, aimed at confirming compliance with specific procedures in the Central Sterilization Department by working personnel, to which the answers are registered in the system and after verification (the system should allow further work or block it)

Systems that manage the circulation of instruments should be consistent with the instrument marking system, e.g., with the Data Matrix code or a comparable or matrix two-dimensional bar code (2D bar code), consisting of black and white fields (modules) placed within the boundaries of the so-called search pattern, in a way that allows the full identification of the instruments in each set and the ability to scan each instrument in the set. In each individual Data Matrix or equivalent code, the encoded information can be placed, e.g., a unique instrument/container number and the ability to use the code for synchronization with IT systems and work organization within the Operational Block and Central Sterilization Department (e.g., composition of surgical instrument sets, circulation within OB/CSD, planning the regeneration and replacement of instruments in sets).

10.6 Intensive medical care area management system

To efficiently manage the entire processes taking place within the hospital, solutions dedicated to particular areas are also created and implemented. An example of advanced software that provides a clinical data repository that stores clinical data is the intensive medical care area management system. It is software designed to collect, store, manipulate, and provide clinical information relevant to the process of providing health care. It should provide users with a broad spectrum of tools to acquire, manipulate, use, and display relevant information to help make accurate, timely, and evidence-based clinical decisions. This type of system creates a complete electronic record of the patient's treatment in the intensive care unit by

- the ability to fully configure the user interface of the system from the level of the administrator application, consisting in the ability to add or hide and remove any functionality, button, and any other element available in the software;
- creating charts of patient's clinical data with division into individual tables presented in separate views and collecting all physiological data from medical devices (presentation in graphical and numerical form).

The system should support processes as part of admission to the ward through the following:

- Review of the complete patient record (including displaying all trends and curves) from previous patient admissions
- Assignment of the bed to the patient
- Documentation of patient's belongings
- Documentation of patient demographics data
- Preliminary assessment of the patient
- Setting physiological goals
- Documentation of patient's home medicines
- Evaluation of patient results
- Documentation of the patient's condition upon arrival, e.g., drains
- Pain assessment
- Laboratory orders

The system should also support processes during ICU stay through the following:

- Current drug management
- Preparation and application of drug doses

- Documentation of care tasks administered to the patient
- Graphic documentation and electronic supervision of the wound healing process
- Adaptation of ventilation
- Monitoring instructions for nursing staff
- Supervision of the balance of liquids based on the interface with automatic calculation of fluid balances
- Daily medical assessments
- Periodic nursing assessments
- Pain assessment
- Documentation of clinical events and incidents
- Documentation of family visits and information provided.

The system should accept (store temporarily) and display DICOM files and provide support for the DICOM standard for archiving, displaying, downloading, and uploading DICOM files. In terms of registration and monitoring the patient, it should enable

- the ability to preregister the patient by filling out the patient identification number, automatically importing personal, clinical, and demographic data from existing records;
- the automatic generation of the ID so that the patient can be assigned to the bed and the data could begin to flow into the patient file;
- the possibility of assigning the patient to the bed on the graphic panel of the ward, reflecting the layout of the room and beds;
- searching for patients by searching for keywords or by means of advanced queries, such as a reference to a specific time interval or a care team. The search should be carried out according to any combination of different elements: patient's name, account number, MR number, date of admission, date of discharge, patient status, transport, ward, care team, bed's number, bed group, bed status.

Personnel should be able to document, analyze, and update diagnoses, problems, interventions, and results of the patient in the primary areas of care: cardiovascular, respiratory, neurological, urological, excretory, temperature, coherence, digestion, skin, mobility, communication, and pain. The system should enable grouping of patients according to selected criteria (e.g., cardiac patients) regardless of place or ward. Choosing a patient from the list should automatically display the full patient chart with a panoramic view of information obtained and presented on a regular basis, such as HR, blood pressure, temperature, reminders, events, planned, and administered medications and other relevant information. A report from any clinically relevant information can be generated and delivered to the admitting unit, such as admission, essential findings, diagnoses, procedures, medicines, and condition during the transfer. The user interface should display spreadsheets presenting graphical and tabular parameter data over time, which are captured by various sources. Data can automatically fill charts using physiological monitors and other medical devices as well as clinical interfaces, such as laboratory and microbiology. Data points can be manually entered or calculated data, such as scoring calculations, and are also displayed in diagrams. Physicians can confirm any data obtained from physiological devices (manually entered values should always be automatically checked). Clinicians can add annotations to any data point, mark it as an error, or mark it with a warning if needed. Each of them has a clear indication on the diagram so that clinicians do not have to seek irregularities. Authorized users can also view parameters for various systems, including respiratory, neurological, temperature, pain, and others, in one tab, allowing an overview of individual patient systems without having to switch to separate views for each of them. Patient's vital parameters are collected from devices automatically and on a regular basis. It is easy to link the patient's vital signs with other patient data, as they are displayed simultaneously over time. Physicians can access and fill any form available in the entire system from a central location without having to look for a chart or button that opens it. They can also view all saved forms, both signed and unsigned, with data for the patient. The system provides a full cycle of treatment and drug management: treatment planning, ordering, reviewing the pharmacy, preparation and administration, reviewing treatment, and reviewing and customizing the order. The system provides easy access to all information necessary to confirm the correctness, for example, administration of any drug because the carer is obliged to check the right patient, the right medicine, the right dose, the right time, and the right route. Nurses or pharmacists can register the preparation of medication doses for the patient. A single dose or multiple doses can be marked as being prepared at once for the patient. Physicians can also mark doses for many patients, just as they were prepared at once. Nurses may perform various activities at doses of defined duration, depending on the dosage status, e.g., they may also undo the validation of a dose that has been incorrectly labeled as being administered. Physicians can order exact doses in exact amounts and at exact times, even for specialist therapies that do not comply with the standard protocol. The system may also recommend replacing the drug and an alternative treatment plan based on hospital policy and support irregular dosing schedules, such as varying doses per day. The system should be equipped with tools to support the doctor's decision, by tracking changes in the patient's condition and deviations from clinical or administrative protocols. The system should inform the doctor about it to cause action by sending on-screen notifications, e-mails about required actions, such as initiating or terminating treatment, activating care protocols, performing tests, or adopting recommended security measures. The system records the event, the conditions that triggered the event, the history of comments, and the validation of each triggered event, and it may inform doctors to consider changing the patient's medicine to a cheaper but equally effective replacement. The system must automatically collect patient monitoring data from cardiac monitors and automatically collect ventilation data from respirators, infusion data from pumps and data from anesthetic machines, data from anesthetic gas analyzers, data from critical parameter analyzers, and other life support devices (graphical and numerical data presentation). On this basis, the system should generate patient reports. Reports can be automatically generated by the end user from the application level after a specific event or according to the schedule (e.g., daily print). The solution must enable the development of a mobile application that fully synchronizes with the software to support nursing documentation, observations, vital signs, drug administration, and task lists for many patients and should guarantee integration with the hospital HIS system together with the delivery and support of necessary operating systems and database systems for the proper functioning of the system.

10.7 Medical device management systems

IT systems supporting medical device management are usually integrated: open ERP systems with functionality, including, among others, management of medical devices; their locations, inspections, contracts, and service calls; and their implementation, including human resources, investment planning, and analysis of the status and value of assets. To improve management procedures, they should provide, among others, functions such as the following:

- User administration (various levels of authorization)
- Management of current failures, periodic inspections, and purchase of spare parts
- Management of already concluded contracts (including lease, lending, purchases, bundled, and test agreements) and cooperation with the contract register system through the ability to attach scans of contracts
- Management of contract features of devices that are required by the payer of medical services
- Editable database of contractors (contact details: companies, individuals, and competence areas)
- Determining the location by linking to inventory systems and the ability to use the data contained therein
- Full functionality of the system available through a web browser (availability of the version for tablet and smartphone)
- Use of the identification data of the equipment already owned by the user—for example, inventory number, bar code, name, model, serial number, year of manufacture, manufacturer, supplier, location, cost center, date of acceptance, last review (with the type of review), last software update, next scheduled review, last repair, warranty period, guarantor, status (deleted, for deletion, in current operation, temporarily decommissioned), type of ownership of the apparatus (lending agreement, ownership, lease, test), service (authorized, alternative, own), and responsible/user (contact details to these people)
- Information on assigning the apparatus to the contract (or multiple contracts) with payers together with the possibility of exporting such data, informing other SU departments about the device being commissioned/decommissioned

- Creating and modifying the classification of devices, technical cards/passports for devices
- The possibility of attaching documents in the .pdf, .jpg, and .bmp format, such as operating manuals, certificates, technical statements (stored on the server, outside the program database, according to a specific scheme also available from the intranet level—without using the application)
- The option of attaching the nameplate as well as the device itself to each device (keeping on the server, outside the database)
- Possibility of attaching links to documents located outside the database on the server, e.g., to the register of contracts
- The ability to filter data by any features, the ability to write filtering schemes (e.g., by cost centers, classification)
- Dedicated application/applet (also mobile) for reporting failures, the need for inspections, etc.
- Possibility of defining users who can submit applications (without limitation as to the amount of software licenses)
- Personal identification: a user with his/her unique ID and password to verify the source of the request, each application registered in the system, the ability to create user groups. Each user with access to strictly defined resources (medical devices) defined on the basis of their affiliation to the selected location
- Defining the minimum registration requirements, e.g., each application must contain at least the following data set: name, type of device, inventory number or another number confirming the possibility of its operation within the unit, location and its availability, cost center, person reporting/responsible person, type of failure, description of failure, telephone, e-mail.
- Automatic sending of a unique notification number, the ability to indicate by the user of the devices only and exclusively from the lists to which the user has permission, e.g., devices assigned to his/her location

To cumulate and organize the stream of information, the system should provide information flow to ensure the continuity of the case and its monitoring at every stage. An exemplary scheme for submitting and maintaining a service case may be the following:
- On the basis of the notification, a task is automatically created, which the administrative person transfers to the own (internal) service or starts the service order procedure (it is also possible to set an automatic redirection)
- Service staff performs tasks based on electronic information; upon completion, they prepare a registered note/report
- Completion of the task is confirmed by the superior of the internal service (it should be possible to issue tasks related to the already executed order, e.g., purchase of parts, additional measurements, or redirect the case to be carried out outside)

- For external orders, the ability to generate, modify, and send price queries to companies from the database and entered manually (additional option to generate a query with a request for a diagnosis valuation)
- Generating orders based on sent offers or based on the information entered
- The ability to generate purchase orders for spare parts for the internal service carried out by own operations
- The possibility of printing a request for proposal and an order adapted to the user's procedures
- Registration of individual stages of the case
- The possibility to take notes to the case
- Circulation of documents regarding the order along with the approvals and comments of the superiors adjusted to the aforementioned hospital procedures
- Automatic report "from review/failure report to completion of effective actions" assigned to the internal service engineer
- Assessment of the service after completion of the intervention
- Registration of the invoice along with costs and connection with the order to verify the legitimacy of costs:
  1. costs of the case—invoice number, date, overall amount, unit amount, the net amount for individual VAT rates
  2. the possibility of breaking the invoice into components, including, at least, the cost of repair, travel, parts
  3. building the history of orders and costs for individual devices from the database.

The task of the system should also be the archiving of orders and the possibility of their analysis and interpretation. To this end, the system should ensure
- archiving and processing of repair information, e.g., costs of repair, costs of used parts and other components affecting the overall cost of repair, and date of completion;
- generating order history along with relevant data: date, contractor, type, and value of materials used;
- the possibility of communication and realization of applications for smartphones/tablets (e.g., preview of orders for a given working group, taking over of orders, execution of orders, adding notes, bar code scanning, entering data on the progress of the case—for authorized users);
- purchase and spare parts registration function purchased and installed directly by technicians/engineers, i.e., the database, in addition to the history of inspections and services, should also include the history of the purchase of spare parts with the assignment of a directly purchased part of the device to which it was purchased;
- alert regarding spare parts held in stock to avoid redundancy of orders;
- creating requests for proposal, offers or orders, or invoices allowing for automatic reading of data from the previous document;

- the possibility of granting varying degrees of authority for selected users, coordinators, and supervisors (e.g., order preview, data entry, and correction, decision making);
- building own templates and sample documents, modification of existing templates during the processing leading to the selection of the contractor, e.g., by the possibility of using more arguments and criteria (not only the price but also other criteria, e.g., qualitative, warranty, technical, economic, related to a contract) to a management decision and with a suitable place for selection argumentation, comments, etc. (documents in electronic form, conducting polemics of negotiation in electronic form, additionally a printout option);
- the possibility of full access to the program by own technical staff, including the ability to generate a direct response to the user, a comment on the status of the repair, waiting time, no possibility of repair, the ability to close orders after completed online work (the required number of licenses in accordance with the number of employees executing orders, the possibility of direct contact with software on the device (smartphone, tablet);
- automatic generation by the system of confirmation of the service performed or information about further use of the device;
- creating technical opinions and deletion opinions, together with the possibility of sending opinions directly to the user and other units of the hospital;
- the registration of invoices, the possibility of accepting electronic invoices and the introduction of processed invoices (scans, other electronic forms), and the ability to easily verify orders versus invoice for cost control;
- creating schedules of medical device reviews according to the given algorithm, e.g., for individual departments, groups of equipment, broken down by time units, and/or costs or according to individual user criteria, informing on the possible aggregation of interventions;
- creating a register of inspections made, including information about the planned date of the next review (the possibility of automatic or individual introduction of deadlines);
- the possibility of marking the type of device review: internal inspection, inspection performed by the external service, and warranty review;
- the ability to define the inspection cycles, in particular, year, half year, quarter, two years, own periods;
- inspection calendars: information about upcoming, exceeding deadlines, completed, canceled, unperformed/unfinished, ended with a negative opinion;
- creating a history of inspections (postwarranty and warranty): in the inspection calendar for all devices covered by the plan, for individual devices, for individual cost centers;
- verifications of appointments and reminder functions:
    a. automatic generation by the program: a reminder, e.g., of the 20th of each month about the devices requiring technical inspection in the following month

    b.   the ability to generate inspection orders for all the devices indicated by the system

    c.   information about exceeded deadlines

- creating within the database a simple search system of devices using ionizing radiation and magnetic field;
- the ability to specify a functional calendar for handling specialist tests of the above-mentioned devices: date of the last test, test result (in the case of negative tests creating noncompliance form (the possibility of circulation of the form along the path proxy–radiological protection inspector–unit manager–department of medical equipment–proxy)–connection with the function of reporting device failures (minimizing documentation);
- the evaluation of the number of devices owned by various criteria: type, model, producer, location, and cost center;
- apparatus replacement value reports for all devices, groups, locations, cost centers, etc.;
- the registration of device operation time and/or device activity;
- the analysis of the technical condition of devices based on

      a.   dates of purchase

      b.   number of operation hours

      c.   numbers of tests

      d.   number and cost of failure and calculation of availability time
- the cost analysis of consumables for individual devices, price change in time, comparison to the competition;
- the introduction of data regarding service contracts/specialist tests—assigning to the contracts the list of devices, duration of the contract, contractors;
- a statement of the operating costs of a given device and for a given group of devices;
- cost statements broken down into cost centers, individual departments, the hospital as a whole: breakdown of costs for failures and inspections, breakdown of costs by places of use, and breakdown of costs by cost centers;
- other cost statements, e.g., related to service contractors, purchase and/or use period, source of purchase (own funds, external financing sources, lent apparatuses, etc.), comparison of service costs for different contractors, at different periods, for different users, comparing the costs of spare parts themselves the same kind;
- cocreating investment and repair plans—generating proposals for a purchase plan based on, among others, the degree of device wear, age, exceeding the profitability ratio of further repairs, the number of available (already owned) devices of the same type and their location, and other set values;
- estimation and evaluation reports of contractors based on, e.g., delays, prices, quality of services, response time: notification—a repair performed and/or completed;
- all reporting in both graphical and numerical form, the ability to generate trend reports;

- importing/exporting data to already functioning programs (financial and accounting, warehouse), the ability to independently modify the structure and content of reports, and the ability to import/export/process numerical data at least in .xls .csv, pdf formats;
- the possibility of cooperation or extension with a module cooperating with RFID systems for the location of devices;
- the automatic preparation of documentation for the receipt of equipment in accordance with the procurement procedure (creation of delivery and acceptance protocols and noncompliance protocols);
- the certification of the service or rejecting damaged/receiving the repaired equipment through the mechanism of the signature on the tablet in the form of graphic notation (or other solution eliminating receipts, confirmations, and other paper documents).

10.8 Radio- and brachytherapy management systems

Examples of management systems that are intended for specialized service of selected facilities are also systems for managing radio- and brachytherapy. The functionality of the software used to manage radiotherapy should provide such activities as
- patient movement management in the radiotherapy, chemotherapy, diagnostics, and surgery units, preparing schedules, and dates of visits;
- identification of patients by means of ID number, photo, and/or bar codes;
- the possibility of introducing external examination results by scanning documents;
- management of clinical trials and automatic adjustment of patients to clinical trials conducted;
- creating procedures for patient management, including chemotherapy, radiotherapy, and surgery;
- remote access to patient data on mobile devices;
- management of the patient portal, enabling conducting surveys, checking dates of visits;
- data exchange between the management system and the irradiation systems in radiotherapy.

Each such system should have its own hardware base based on a central data exchange server providing data exchange with external devices in the DICOM standard, data exchange about patients with HIS hospital system in the HL7 protocol, and automatic backup and data archiving tools. For direct work with the system, the following tools are used: direct management systems in radiotherapy, chemotherapy, diagnostics, and surgery units; control stations in therapeutic devices (min 2 for each irradiating device) and in the rooms of diagnostic equipment (min 1 station for each device); medical stations with medical monitors in consultation rooms; a review station with a projector and preview monitors in the consulting room; management stations in treatment planning rooms and additional devices such as scanners for medical records; bar code readers (for each management position and at each diagnostic and therapeutic devices); or barcode printers for each management station.

In turn, the 3D treatment planning system for brachytherapy is a system that allows manual and automatic preparation of contours for target and critical areas when planning brachytherapy treatment. It is a tool for the preparation of plans and 3D distribution enabling planning for stationary photon and electron beams, dose calculations, and presentation of results in the form of dose-volume histograms. In addition, it should provide the following features:

- Automatic and manual application of various series of images: CT, NMR, and PET
- Exchange of image data with external devices in the DICOM standard
- Exchange of data on patients with an HIS hospital system in the HL7 protocol
- Automatic backup and data archiving tools
- Transfer of the treatment plan of the offered planning system directly to the HDR camera via a computer network
- Import of teleradiotherapeutic 3D treatment plans from other treatment planning systems to offered DICOM RT brachytherapy planning stations
- Summing of teletherapeutic plans (imported in the DICOM RT standard from other 3D treatment planning systems) with brachytherapy plans made on the brachytherapy planning stations offered
- The possibility of planning brachytherapy based on 2D images from a radiotherapy simulator or C-Arm X-ray apparatus
- Planning 3D brachytherapy based on CT images from a computer tomograph and using NMR images
- 3D fusion of CT and NMR images and overlapping of two different sets of images (e.g., CT and NMR)
- Presentation of 3D absorbed dose schedules and presentation of 2D absorbed dose schedules in any plane
- 3D display of the patient along with the contoured structures, reconstructed applicators and CT images
- Manual or automatic reconstruction of catheters
- User selection of the average electron density for inhomogeneity correction (to remove the contrast of the material or image artifact)
- Optimization of the dose distribution by means of graphic mouse modeling of the 3D isodose shape and functions to optimize the location of the source based on the set dose values in the 3D structures of the patient

Computer equipment for the offered 3D brachytherapy planning software, as well as any other system, should be offered and operated in a configuration compatible with the requirements of the manufacturer of the offered system.

Tomasz Rogula, Aneta Myszka, Tanawat Vongsurbchart, and Nasit Vurgun

11 Robotic surgery training, simulation, and data collection

11.1 History and progress of training in minimally invasive surgery

Minimally invasive surgery, done either robotically or laparoscopically, has many advantages over traditional open surgery when performed successfully. These include fewer or smaller incisions, decreased blood loss, less pain, reduced infection, reduced scarring, and potentially shorter hospitalizations with faster recovery times for patients.

Among minimally invasive surgery types, laparoscopy is by far the most common. The term *laparoscopy* refers to procedures performed inside the abdomen and pelvis, using special surgical tools and a camera. These are placed into the patient through small incisions where trocars are placed. The trocars serve as pivots and points of reference for the laparoscopic instruments. The body cavity is usually insufflated with CO_2 gas, to allow more room for manipulations. Laparoscopic techniques feature prominently in general surgery, gynecology, and urology. Examples of laparoscopic procedures done by general surgeons include appendectomy, cholecystectomy, esophageal surgery, gastric surgery, colorectal surgery, liver surgery, adrenalectomy, pancreatectomy, splenectomy, and hernia repair, to name a few.

To facilitate surgeon training in laparoscopy, the American Board of Surgery (ABS) implemented the Fundamentals of Laparoscopic Surgery (FLS) training course in 2008 as a mandatory prerequisite for the ABS certifying exam. The FLS curriculum was implemented by the Society of American Gastrointestinal and Endoscopic Surgeons (SAGES) in 1999, designed to teach the fundamental knowledge and technical skills required for basic laparoscopy in a standardized and systematic manner [1]. The cognitive component consists of preoperative considerations, intraoperative considerations, basic laparoscopic procedures, and postoperative considerations, which are presented in the way of didactic modules. Meanwhile, the hands-on component consists of exercises that teach bimanual dexterity through tasks involving the manipulation of objects inside a training box physical simulation environment. The FLS manual tasks are peg transfer, precision cutting, ligating loop placement, suture with extracorporeal knot, and suture with intracorporeal knot. Each task has objective benchmarks of efficiency and precision, obtained from experts, as well as defined errors with penalties, which trainees should learn to avoid [1]. Upon completion of the FLS skills-based training curriculum, which on average takes about 10 hours of distributed learning through numerous repetitions of each task, surgeon candidates then complete a high-stakes examination where they must demonstrate standardized levels of proficiency to obtain FLS certification [2].

Robotic surgery, also known as robot-assisted surgery, differs from laparoscopy in a number of ways. First of all, it restores some of the visuospatial deficit that is lost in laparoscopy, through 3D stereoscopic visualization. Second, there are additional features that can be desirable for the surgeon, including tremor filtering, eye tracking, and navigation, which can enable the surgeon to be more precise, while potentially saving valuable time intraoperatively in the operating room (OR). One downside to robotic surgery, besides the much higher cost of purchase and maintenance, is the longer set up time, also known as docking time, when compared with laparoscopy. Readers should also recognize that the number of FDA-approved surgical robotic devices available on the market is very limited thus far, when compared with the ubiquitous number of FDA-approved laparoscopic tools and instruments, which are readily available on the market for surgeons or healthcare facilities to purchase and use (Figs. 11.1 and 11.2).

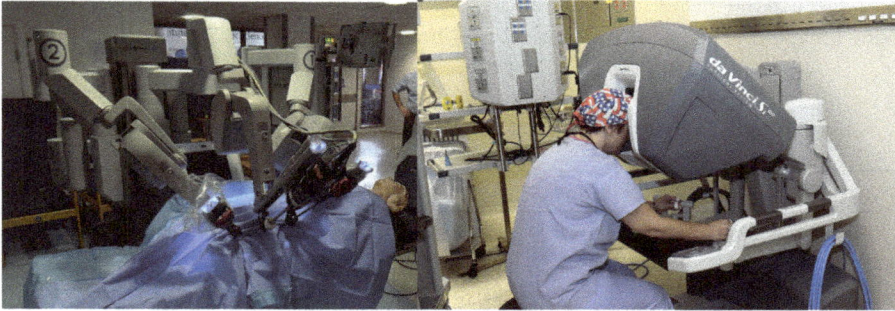

Fig. 11.1: da Vinci Surgical Robot. Left image credit: Creative Commons 3.0 Unported License, Photo taken by: cmglee, WikiMedia Commons. https://commons.wikimedia.org/wiki/File:Cmglee_Cambridge_Science_ Festival_2015_da_Vinci.jpg. Right image credit: US Army, taken by: Jeff L Troth https://www.army.mil/article/152941/robotic_da_vinci_arrives_at_evans.

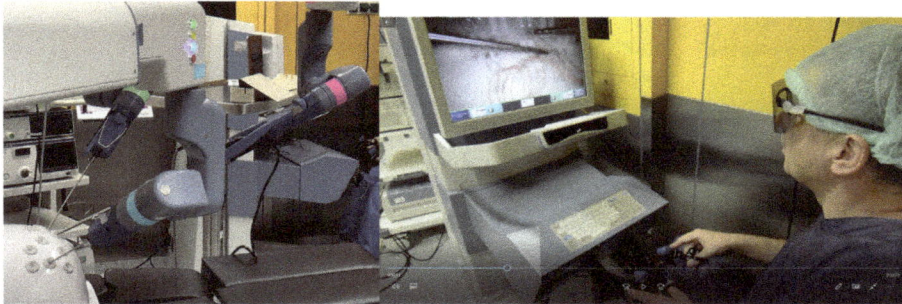

Fig. 11.2: Senhance Surgical Robot. Photo credit: own work.

The best known, most widely used, and most mature surgical robotic device on the world market is the da Vinci surgical robotic system from Intuitive Surgical Inc. Approved by the FDA in 2000, it held a monopoly share of the robotic surgery market and had virtually no competitor until the Senhance surgical robotic system from TransEnterix, formerly known as the Telelap ALF-X, which obtained FDA approval in 2017. Although other surgical robots with FDA approval exist, besides the da Vinci and the Senhance, they are not used for the purposes of general surgery. Specialized surgical domains with FDA-approved surgical robots include colonoscopy, catheter insertion, transoral surgery, and bronchoscopy. A review of current and emerging surgical robotic systems can be found in the 2019 review by Peters et al. [3] (Tab. 11.1).

Another significant difference between laparoscopy and robotic surgery is the fact that a standardized and accredited education curriculum for robotic surgery is still lacking. The most developed training program so far is the Fundamentals of Robotic Surgery (FRS) curriculum. The FRS was created with the goal of teaching the common set of skills to operate with robotic surgery devices [4]. However, it is worth noting that the curriculum was mainly built around the da Vinci surgical system because of its pioneer role in the introduction of robotic surgery, being the only FDA-approved robotic device for general surgical procedures and holding a monopoly share of the market

Tab. 11.1: Selected list of FDA-approved robotic surgery systems [3]

Device Name	Manufacturer	Surgery Types	Notable Features
da Vinci surgical robotic system	Intuitive Surgical	Laparoscopy, urology, gynecology, thoracoscopy	Tremor filtering
Senhance surgical robotic system	TransEnterix	Laparoscopy, gynecology	Haptic feedback, eye tracking, fully reusable instruments
FLEX robotic system	Medrobotics Corp	Transoral, pharyngeal, laryngeal	Telescopic instruments
SPIDER—single port instrument delivery	TransEnterix	Laparoscopy	Triangulation of instruments from port
NeoGuide Colonoscope	Intuitive Surgical	Colonoscopy	3D mapping
Invendoscopy E200 for colonoscopy	Invendo Medical GmbH	Colonoscopy	Sterile, single-use
FreeHand camera control system for laparoscopy	Freehand 2010 Ltd.	Laparoscopy	Laser guided
Sensei X surgical robot for cardiac catheter placement	Hansen Medical	Cardiac catheterization	Navigation, haptic feedback
Monarch Platform for bronchoscopy	Auris Health	Bronchoscopy	Navigation, user-friendly controller

since its release in 2000. The FRS curriculum is described in detail in Chapter 11.2. For the Senhance surgical system, a specific training program or simulation platform does not yet exist, although it was made to mimic traditional laparoscopy, unlike the da Vinci robot. This raises the very interesting research question of whether laparoscopic skills will be transferable to the newly FDA-approved Senhance robot, and how that might affect the learning curve for trainees. Our group is presently conducting a research study to answer this question.

The lack of a nonstandardized and nonaccredited curriculum raises concerns for patients, and regulatory bodies about whether surgeons are sufficiently trained to perform surgeries with these emerging technologies. The regulatory body responsible for the manufacturing, performance, and safety of medical devices is the FDA. According to the FDA, robotically assisted surgery is both safe and effective, when used by surgeons who have adequate training [5]. However, the FDA does not regulate or standardize the practice of medicine and physician training. Instead, the FDA views training, development, and implementation of medical devices as a responsibility of manufacturers, physicians, and health care facilities. It also argues for the role of professional bodies and specialty board organizations, such as the ABS, in regulating the training of physicians. The FDA further advises physicians and workplaces to ensure that all staff have adequate training and credentialing so that robotically assisted surgical devices (RASD) can be used safely and efficaciously. The concerns of the FDA regarding training and credentialing were recently made public, in a 2019 press release, cautioning patients and healthcare providers on the safe use of surgical robotic systems in breast cancer surgery [6]. In the article, the FDA clearly states that the RASD were approved for general use on the grounds of safety and efficacy, citing that insufficient evidence currently exists on whether these devices influence survival outcomes for patients undergoing oncologic surgeries such as mastectomy. The FDA therefore recommends that a common sense approach be taken when adopting this new technology, where adequate discussion with the patient must take place, with respect to the benefits, risks, and alternatives to doing such a surgery robotically.

Our aim in writing this book chapter was to review the current state of the art in robotic surgery simulation and training and to give readers the viewpoint of the surgeon, so that readers can explore and work on robotic surgery problems without losing sight of the needs of the surgeon, who after all is the end user for these exciting, new technologies. Readers are encouraged to further explore other recent reviews on the topic of robotic surgery devices, training, and simulation [3, 7–11]. In addition, readers may obtain the summary report from the Institution for Surgical Excellence: Robotic Registry consensus Conference from September 2016, which provides a comprehensive analysis of the state of robotic surgery, with lists of expert recommendations toward implementing systemwide quality improvement measures and data collection frameworks to facilitate future progress in robotic surgery [12].

11.2 Simulation and training with respect to robotic surgery

11.2.1 Training

Training in robotic surgery is a natural progression. Starting from basic or rather simple tasks, the trainee must learn to manipulate objects purposefully through increasingly difficult and novel ways, while using only their eyes, hands, and other unnatural modes of computer guidance for feedback. For this reason, completing a basic task from open surgery, such as making one suture or one knot, can require significantly greater levels of concentration, dexterity, and experience to perform successfully using a surgical robotic system. From our experience, trainees in robotic surgery also start at different baselines and report different levels of subjective stress during the training process. Psychological demand, physical demand, time pressure, performance anxiety, effort, and frustration all contribute to the overall learning experience and robotic education of the trainees.

To master any surgical skill, the trainee must be present and persistent for regular training to take place. In addition, the learner must have access through the institution to a conducive learning environment where they can practice tasks without distraction, and with enough time allocated to dedicated learning until a desired level of competence and proficiency can be reached.

In reality, the progression in training starts with acquiring basic knowledge about robotic surgery (for example, through e-learning from the Internet), and with assistance in set up during a robotic surgery operation (this is referred to as a bedside assistant) [11]. Learning is supplemented by the observation of robotic surgeries in the OR or behind the surgeon on the console, although observation can also take the form of virtual reality (VR) learning platforms such as GIBLIB, or emerging augmented reality technologies such as the Microsoft HoloLens 2.

Simulation is the next logical step in learning, which starts with console controls and the completion of basic motor tasks. Beyond this stage, the trainee moves on to complete a series of simulator modules, of increasing difficulty and requiring increasing levels of dexterity and coordination. This stage is thought to assume a classical learning curve, where early gains are achieved relatively quickly, but mastery requires exponential amounts of time spent training.

As the trainee becomes more competent on simulator tasks requiring increased levels of mastery and demonstrates increased proficiency with reference to the expert, they can progress safely to clinical tasks, which require substantially more responsibility than simulators. The training then takes place on patients, either through dual-console trainers, or through assisting on cases with the console with the help of an expert robotic surgeon, who is stationed physically in the OR or who provides telementoring off-site.

Altogether, training follows evidence-based simulation methods, synthesized into standardized robotic surgery training programs, such as the FRS, made by expert robotic surgeon groups who have a stake in educating medical students, residents, fellows, colleagues, and successors. Currently, there does not exist any learning modules whose completion and credentialing is regulated or required by the ABS, which oversees surgeon training.

11.2.2 Simulation

Simulation is an essential educational learning ground that allows for interactive training to take place in an environment that recreates or mimics real-world scenarios. The goals of this type of training can vary, but most simulators aim to teach specific skills that can be taught in clinical or preclinical simulation environments. No matter how realistic a simulator can be, it is not identical to real clinical cases with real patients [13]. Therefore, most simulator training takes place in the initial "preclinical" learning phase because the simulation purpose is to ensure that a sufficient amount of practice has taken place before trainees can use the technology to perform similar tasks on real patients. Therefore, simulators are used to improve surgeon performance within a safe and controlled training environment where the critical steps of any surgical operation may be recreated and practiced without requiring a patient.

There are several simulators available on the market for robotic surgery training [14]. Training products are generally classified into two categories: mechanical simulators and VR simulators. The former group consists of a physical training box, whereas the latter group provides a virtual training environment that is specially designed to mimic real-world tasks.

11.2.3 VR simulators

A summary of VR simulator platforms, which are presently used for robotic surgery training, can be found in Tab. 11.2. Readers wishing to read at length the detailed features of each simulation system should refer to Peters et al. [3]. The usefulness of a simulator depends on its capability to test the criteria that it is designed to evaluate, which is called *validity* [18]. The simulators mentioned in the table have demonstrated evidence of face validity (has real-life resemblance), content validity (mimics testing conditions), and construct validity (can differentiate novices from experts) [17, 19–24]. The da Vinci Skills Simulator (dVSS) and the ProMIS simulator require the application of the da Vinci robot to train, whereas the other simulators are stand-alone systems and do not require the da Vinci robot system to train. It is worth mentioning that the ProMIS system is a unique, hybrid VR and physical simulation training box system. ProMIS is attached to the da Vinci and presents the trainee with a more familiar, laparoscopic user interface.

Tab. 11.2: List of simulators and training features [3, 10, 15–17]

VR Simulator Platform	Company and Year of Release	Description of Training Exercises	Scoring Criteria
da Vinci Skills Simulator (dVSS)	Intuitive Surgical, 2011	Console controls training, EndoWrist manipulations, clutch use, camera control, electrosurgery (coagulation, dissection, cutting), needle exercises, suturing exercises, knot tying, games, complete surgical procedures	Task completion time, economy of motion, object drops, instrument out-of-view, use of excess force, radius of sphere centered on instrument tip, instrument collisions, and overall composite score
dV-Trainer (dVT)	Mimic, 2007	Console controls training, EndoWrist manipulations, clutch use, camera control, electrosurgery (coagulation, dissection, cutting), needle exercises, suturing exercises, knot tying, games	Task completion time, economy of motion, object drops, instrument out-of-view, use of excess force, radius of sphere centered on instrument tip, instrument collisions, and overall composite score
Robotic Surgery Simulator	Simulated Surgical Systems, 2010	Console controls training, visuospatial manipulation, needle exercises, electrosurgery, fourth arm control, tissue and vessel dissection, video-guided surgical training assisted by haptic feedback, complete surgical procedures	Task completion time, object drops, bimanual reporting of instruments out-of-view, bimanual reporting of grasps, camera movement optimization, object drops, use of excess force on tissue, instrument collisions, and overall composite score
RobotiX Mentor	3D Systems, 2014	Similar to dVSS training but with on-screen step-by-step coaching, FRS physical dome exercises with increasing difficulty, RTN and FLS-based skills training, single-site instrument suturing, stapler training, complete surgical procedures	Task completion time, bimanual reporting of instruments out-of-view, bimanual movement counts and path length, bimanual reporting of collisions, camera movement optimization, number of clutch uses
ProMIS	Haptica, 2003	Laparoscopic manipulations, needle handling, suturing	Completion time, path length, smoothness of motion

11.2.4 Physical training

In addition to VR simulator training, trainees can improve their robotic surgery skills using physical simulators, which can be further split into dry lab and wet lab flavors.

Dry lab trainers typically make use of synthetic materials which can be as simple as spherical beads or shoelaces, to highly detailed and realistic organlike phantoms from materials that are designer made to mimic biological tissue. These trainers can teach real-life surgical skills such as grasping, cutting, and suturing and robot-specific skills such as camera control and clutch use.

Wet lab, on the other hand, typically uses cadaveric human or animal tissues (fresh or frozen) for a more realistic simulation experience. In addition to all of the skills that can be practiced upon in dry lab, wet lab simulations can be used to teach electrocautery with energy devices, in an environment where interaction of surgical robot instruments with biological tissues is nearly identical to what the surgeon would experience during a real case. Animal tissues are generally favored over cadaveric tissues. Although performing operations on live animals is occasionally done, it is rather uncommon unless there is a very good reason to anesthetize and euthanize such an animal for the purposes of surgical training.

Lastly, box trainers that are available for laparoscopy can be adapted for use in robotic surgery. Examples of box trainers from laparoscopy that have been adapted to robotic surgery include the FLS trainer, which is the gold standard across the United States [25], and the Laparo trainer, which is a popular and cost-effective option, particularly in the European Union. The reason for this modification is that the laparoscopic box ports likely will not readily accommodate the robotic surgery instrument arms.

11.3 Robotic courses

Although many simulators were released and have been implemented in training surgeons on robotic surgery, proper training courses, criteria, and credentialing guidelines are still in the early phase of development. Currently, the leading robotic surgery training program is the FRS.

11.3.1 Fundamentals of robotic surgery

FRS is an educational, training, and assessment robotic surgical skill program [26], available online at frsurgery.org. The consensus conference began the development of FRS program [4, 27] funded by the Department of Defense and Intuitive Surgical System [26]. Professionals of different areas including behavioral psychologists, medical educators, statisticians, psychometricians, and over 80 national/international robotic surgery experts were involved in establishing the FRS curriculum through the use of the full life cycle development process [28]. Essentially, FRS was developed to be generalized to any robotic surgical systems and not limited to da Vinci surgical system [27]. Pioneers in robotic surgery cooperated together during four consensus conferences to produce the final FRS curriculum, which is composed of four modules with seven psychomotor skills tasks [8] that would be assessed based on the agreed upon 25 criteria of robotic surgery, listed in Tab. 11.3. FRS validation was completed in 2016 through a multi-institutional, multispecialty, randomized controlled trial [27].

The FRS curriculum consists of four online modules, listed in Tab. 11.4. Each module consists of short narrated video lectures with a quiz at the end of each module [29].

Tab. 11.3: Consensus criteria for the evaluation of FRS trainees [7, 4, 12]

Preoperative	Intraoperative	Postoperative
1. Situation awareness	9. Closed loop communication	24. Undocking
2. Instrument-hand-eye coordination	10. Docking	25. Transition to bedside assist
3. Needle driving	11. Knot tying	
4. Atraumatic handling	12. Instrument exchange	
5. Safety of operating field	13. Suture handling	
6. Camera controls	14. Energy sources	
7. Clutch use	15. Cutting	
8. Blunt and sharp dissection	16. Foreign body management	
	17. Ergonomic position	
	18. Wrist articulation	
	19. Robotic trocars	
	20. System setting	
	21. Multiarm control	
	22. Operating room setup	
	23. Respond to robot system error	

Tab. 11.4: FRS modules

Module 1: Introduction to Surgical Robotic Systems	Introduction to minimally invasive surgery, components of robotic system, and system functionality
Module 2: Didactic Instruction for Robotic Surgery Systems	Instructions for safe and effective use of robotic procedures in the preoperative, intraoperative, and postoperative phases [8]
Module 3: Psychomotor Skills Curriculum	Description of the physical model of the FRS dome (fig of the dome), description and scoring guidelines for the seven tasks
Module 4: Team Training and Communication Skills	Communication training for surgical teams, consisting checklists during preop, docking, intraop and postop phases, as well as modules on situational awareness, teamwork, and mutual support

11.3.2 Robotics Training Network (RTN)

'The Robotics Training Network is a multi-center training network, formed in 2010, which oversees the structured training of surgeons in robotic surgery, requiring the completion of a validation tool to assess robot-assisted surgery proficiency [30]. It consists of three phases: bedside assistance, surgeon console training, and maintenance of learning skills. In 2011, the RTN had settled an accredited curriculum of best practices in robot-assisted surgery among its academic institution partners. The RTN curriculum has three phases, detailed in Tab. 11.5 [30].

Tab. 11.5: Phases of training in robotic training network [30]

Phase I (bedside assistance)	Self-guided learning using online materials and quizzes, a dry lab and simulator, and an OR component. In addition, there are problem solving, professionalism, and communication components.
Phase II (surgeon console)	Dry labs must be completed before trainees can proceed to the OR.
Phase III (in development)	Ongoing maintenance of skills

As of 2013, the RTN has been introduced to 50 programs to develop or evaluate outcome measures, curricula, and validation studies and to improve patient safety and quality of care [30]. Robot-assisted skills are assessed using the Robotic-Objective Structured Assessment of Technical Skills, which measures performance on tasks based on depth perception and accuracy, force in tissue handling, dexterity, and efficiency. This assessment has demonstrated construct validity [26].

11.3.3 SAGES Robotics Masters Series

The Robotics Masters Series (RMS) is a training program from SAGES, which is a combination of e-learning modules and on-site learning, taking place at annual conferences for a fee. The curriculum features three stages of difficulty and achievement: competency, proficiency, and master [31]. RMS completion at the competency level of achievement is deemed to be approximately equal to what a graduating general surgery chief resident should be able to achieve. Proficiency achievement is the next level, which is approximately equivalent to what a junior surgeon, a few years out of training, should be able to achieve. Lastly, master level of achievement is the highest achievement in RMS and approximates to what an experienced surgeon should be able to achieve after many years of surgery practice [31]. Each training level incorporates didactics (recorded videos and lecture learning) and robotic surgery skill training (simulation and cadaver training) but also includes mentorship [31].

11.3.4 Fundamental skills of robot-assisted surgery (FSRS) training program

The FSRS is an on-site robotic surgery training program from the Applied Technology Lab for Advanced Surgery (ATLAS) in Roswell Park Comprehensive Cancer Center, established in 2007. What began as an initiative to improve safety and quality with respect to robotic surgery systems transformed into a validated learning program with on-site training center, employing collaboration of surgeon experts and developers of VR systems [32, 33].

The training program contains four modules spanning from basic to advanced (state of performance) levels of achievement and lasting between a few days to a few weeks. The VR simulator that is used is the dVSS, but in addition to exercises specific to this system, a combination of dry lab and wet lab simulations is also practiced by trainees. Lastly, the training program incorporates parts of the FLS curriculum, perhaps because ATLAS is a partner institution of SAGES.

To give trainees real-world practical experience, FSRS bridges simulation training with hands-on tutorial training by nonphysician experts on machine docking and troubleshooting. Lastly, FSRS trainees observe live cases in robotic surgery [33]. A full description of the training is beyond the scope of this book chapter, but it can be found on the FSRS Web site for interested readers.

11.3.5 da Vinci Technology Training Pathway

The da Vinci Technology Training Pathway is an online training course created by Intuitive Surgical Inc. that accompanies the da Vinci surgical robot system [34]. Surgical worksheets and guides are provided in this portal to assist the users with their training. There are four phases of the training program described in the Tab. 11.6 [35].

Tab. 11.6: da Vinci Technology Training Pathway [35]

Phase I: Introduction to da Vinci Technology	Test drive the da Vinci Surgical System
	Review procedure video relevant to your planned da Vinci procedures
	Complete live epicenter and/or standard case observation
	Complete live standard case observation
Phase II: da Vinci Technology Training	Complete da Vinci Technology online training (recommended)
	Complete da Vinci Technology In-Service with da Vinci representative
	Complete da Vinci Technology online assessment
	Perform da Vinci Technology Skills Drills
	– Skills Drills
	– Skills SimulatorTM (if available)
	Review two full-length procedure videos relevant to your planned da Vinci procedures on da Vinci Online Community
	Complete preparation for da Vinci Technology Training (all above prerequisites must be completed before attendance)

Tab.11.6 (Continued)

	Schedule and attend da Vinci Technology Training
	Important: da Vinci Technology Training is either 1 or 2 days, dependent on clinical specialty. Training times are dependent on the training center's hours of operation. Please contact your da Vinci representative for start and end times.
	− If an attendee is more than 30 minutes late, the training may be cancelled and no certificate awarded.
	− Leaving the training event before the completion of all tasks will result in no certificate being awarded.
	− The surgeon is responsible for all costs associated with rescheduling when the reschedule is due to tardiness or early departure.
	− If the surgeon is unable to complete the protocol within the scheduled time, no certificate will be awarded; however, rescheduling to complete another full da Vinci Technology Training will be permitted at no cost to the surgeon.
Phase III: Initial Case Series Plan	Complete initial case series
	Complete two da Vinci Technology skills activities per week, for example:
	− assist in a da Vinci procedure
	− perform a da Vinci procedure
	− complete a da Vinci Technology Skills Drills session
	− complete a da Vinci Skills Simulator session (if available)
	− review a da Vinci Surgery procedure video relevant to your planned da Vinci procedures
Phase IV: Continuing Development	Attend surgeon-led course(s) (Course details are available in the da Vinci Training Passport brochure and course catalog. If not available in your market, please check with your da Vinci representative for course details.)
	Complete at least two additional activities after initial case series:
	− Surgeon lecture program
	− Complex da Vinci procedure observation
	− Complex da Vinci procedure video review
	− da Vinci surgery webinar
	− Peer-to-peer consultation via Surgical Congress

11.4 Early clinical training in robotic surgery

Mentoring is a type of training whereby the learner is supervised and guided by a more experienced surgeon. It can be especially useful in the second part of the training process, after the trainee has acquired competence in basic skills and knowledge. Although simulators make up the majority of training time for residents and fellows, the content validity of simulators of current technologies still cannot represent all real-world possibilities. Actual physical limitations or unforeseen events can happen during any procedure in the OR. Hence, as the user gains competency, the next best step in training takes place during real, clinical procedures.

The da Vinci Model Si provides dual-console capability for junior and supervising surgeons to operate at the same time and transfer the control to and from each other during the operation [36]. This allows the mentoring surgeon to guide the trainee at specific points in each procedure, for example, during suturing. This controller-swap mode has improved the learning curve and lessened the anxiety of the trainee during the early stages of clinical training [37]. The term "telementoring" has been assigned to this way of supervision.

11.5 Global data collection for robotic surgery

The exponential increase in information that is now generated by RASD warrants the need to standardize data collection, storage, and sharing practices. A global robotic surgery registry that collects, stores, and facilitates high-quality information flow could have many potential benefits for surgeons, regulators, hospitals, and robotic device manufacturers. For example, surgeons or trainees could obtain real-time feedback on their operative performance, such as on the economy and efficiency of their movements. Regulators or licensing bodies could use the registry to improve existing training programs and for establishing benchmarks for certification, credentialing, and continuing education purposes. Hospitals could search for patient outcomes and develop processes that enhance the quality of care, optimize workflow, and reduce the costs associated with robotic surgery. Lastly, manufacturers could conduct pre- and postmarketing surveillance of their devices and identify areas for future innovation.

In 2016, the Robotic Registry Consensus Conference was organized, which brought together experts and decision makers from healthcare, government, and industry, with the goal of organizing a national robot-assisted surgery registry [12]. The consensus opinion was that a registry should be constructed, and that it should meet the following criteria: open to the collection of data from all RASD procedures across all specialties, analyze and process data in near real time, collect data that are crucial for distinguishing between device-related malfunctions versus non-device-related events, prevent duplicate data entry, and serve as a resource to participating institutions for evaluating patient safety, and for surgeons to use for self-assessment and self-improvement.

During the conference, three separate working groups created guidelines for data and reports, which ought to be collected from all robotic surgical devices [12]. A second goal of the meeting was to link device data with clinical outcomes obtained from partner institutions. Through this integration, it may be possible to tell in the future whether a poor outcome is linked to device malfunction or perhaps to surgeons and hospital teams who may not have had adequate training with the device. In either case, the goal of the registry is to generate evidence that can then be used to improve healthcare processes and patient outcomes. The consensus recommendations from these working groups are summarized in Tab. 11.7–11.9.

Tab. 11.7: Group 1 structure and metrics for current data repositories [12]

Device malfunction	– System error codes and faults – Loss of video – System transferred into a recoverable or nonrecoverable safety state – Display of blurry images at surgeon's console or assistant's touch screen – Burnt/broken parts and components – Fell into surgical field or body cavity
Generic surgeon errors	Visceral injury: – burn/puncture/avulsion/transection – number of reversible/nonreversible complications Device use errors: – collision of arms – pedal confusion – off-site injury/lack of device visualization
Case descriptors	– Time of surgery/time of day/faults – Level of surgeon experience – Demographics of team training – Approach (e.g., hybrid) – Emergency versus elective – Alerts (improper/not enough)
Team-based errors	– Inadequate experience with handling emergency situations – Lack of training with specific system features – Inadequate troubleshooting of technical problem/system/instrument checks before procedure – Incorrect port placements/docking errors/electrocautery settings

Tab. 11.8: Group 2 consensus on measurement data collection for RSDR [12]

Desirable data [38]	Categories of collected data: – Discharge with comorbidities and procedures – Cancer stage or some disease – Discharge disposition – Length of stay – Reoperation – Anesthesia time
Available databases	NSQIP STS SGO SAGES AHSQC NCDB
Limitations of data collection	– Patients do not come back to the same hospital – Linkage with claims can validate whether sicker patients return to the same or other hospital – MACRA will require return to same provider

Tab. 11.9: Group 3 consensus on the implementation of RSDR [12]

Data the robotic systems are capable of "reporting"	– System make/model
	– Time and date of procedure
	– Surgeon ID instruments selection
	– Time stamps of all reported events (automated)
	– Maintenance history
	– Accidental actuation
	– Deviation from plan (robot specific)
	– How often a feature is used (workflow)
	– Ergonomic indicators
	– Camera specification and manipulation
	– Surgeon engagement time at the console
	– Total OR time/case time/console time
	– Energy and setting of energy device
	– Energy use history
	– Insufflator time and amount of gas used
	– Inputs to the instruments
	– Power source errors
	– Robotic arm failure
	– Registration error (robot specific)
Data facilitated from sources outside the device	– Surgeon profile/experience/glove size
	– Cloud source of video and audio
	– Tissue condition
	– Procedure type
	– Inform verification spec
	– Was it used as intended
	– Automatically collected data
	– Manual time stamps
Future concerns	– Cloud sourcing data
	– Hardware/software malfunction
	– Robotic coordinator or industry rep entering data
Training issues	– FRS or FLS should be completed to validate the use of the device
	– Maintenance of certification on the device

In summary, data collection in robotic surgery is a work in progress. The Coordinated Registry Network (CRN) for RASD is currently under construction and will most likely be available for access through MDEpiNet in late 2020 [39]. In the future, this CRN and others like it will facilitate real-time data collection from RASD for marketing surveillance, evidence generation, and regulatory decision making. However, registry technologies are still in the early phase, and infrastructure differences between large and small healthcare institutions will likely remain an obstacle to the widespread adoption and use of this technology. The National Evaluation System for health Technology Coordinating Center is working closely with the FDA to accelerate the construction of registries that will link clinical data, billing records, and health records with device data [40]. The final proposal for integration and data flow is shown in Fig. 11.3, which

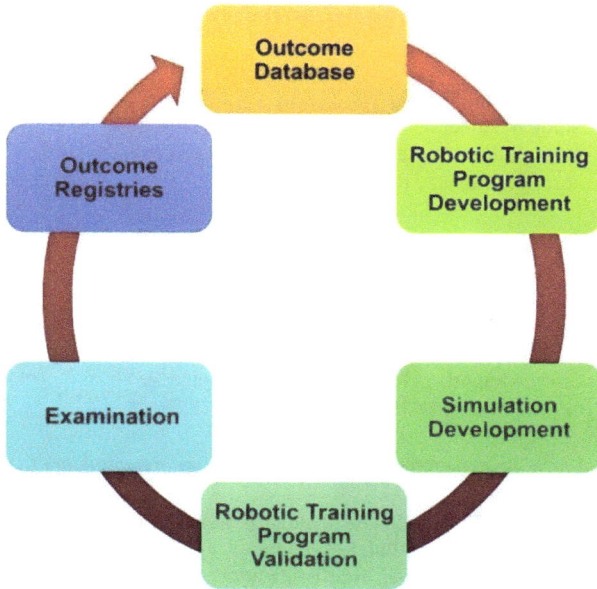

Fig. 11.3: Full cycle model of dataflow for robotic technologies.

depicts a cycle of continuous improvement in robotic surgery based on registry evidence and clinical outcomes.

11.6 References

[1] Tsuda S. "Fundamentals of laparoscopic surgery—a SAGES Wiki article." SAGES, www.sages. org/wiki/fundamentals-laparoscopic-surgery/ (accessed July 1, 2019).
[2] Ritter EM, Scott DJ. "Design of a proficiency-based skills training curriculum for the fundamentals of laparoscopic surgery." *Surgical Innovation* 14, no. 2 (2007): 107–2.
[3] Peters BS, Armijo PR, Krause C, et al. "Review of emerging surgical robotic technology." *Surgical Endoscopy* 32 (2018): 1636. https://doi.org/10.1007/s00464-018-6079-2.
[4] Smith R, Patel V, Satava R. "Fundamentals of robotic surgery: a course of basic robotic surgery skills based upon a 14-society consensus template of outcomes measures and curriculum development." *International Journal of Medical Robotics and Computer Assisted Surgery* 10, no. 3 (2013): 379–84. doi:10.1002/rcs.1559.
[5] Center for Devices and Radiological Health. *Computer-Assisted Surgical Systems*. U.S. Food and Drug Administration. https://www.fda.gov/medical-devices/surgery-devices/computer-assisted-surgical-systems (published March 13, 2019; accessed July 3, 2019).
[6] Center for Devices and Radiological Health. *Caution Using Robotically-Assisted Surgical Devices in Women's Health*. U.S. Food and Drug Administration. https://www.fda.gov/medical-devices/safety-communications/caution-when-using-robotically-assisted-surgical-devices-womens-health-including-mastectomy-and (published February 27, 2019; accessed July 3, 2019).

[7] Rogula T, Acquafresca PA, Bazan M. "Training and credentialing in robotic surgery." In *Essentials of Robotic Surgery*, edited by Kroh M, Chalikonda S. Cham: Springer, 2015.

[8] George EI, Smith R, Levy JS, Brand TC. "Simulation in robotic surgery." In *Comprehensive Healthcare Simulation: Surgery and Surgical Subspecialties*, edited by Stefanidis D, Korndorffer J Jr., Sweet R. Cham: Springer, 2019.

[9] Bric, JD, Lumbard DC, Frelich MJ, et al. "Current state of virtual reality simulation in robotic surgery training: a review." *Surgical Endoscopy* 30 (2016): 2169. https://doi.org/10.1007/s00464-015-4517-y.

[10] MacCraith E, Forde JC, Davis NF. "Robotic simulation training for urological trainees: a comprehensive review on cost, merits and challenges." *Journal of Robotic Surgery* (2019). doi:10.1007/s11701-019-00934-1.

[11] Sridhar AN, Briggs TP, Kelly JD, Nathan S. "Training in robotic surgery—an overview." *Current Urology Reports* 18, no. 8 (2017). doi:10.1007/s11934-017-0710-y.

[12] Robotic Registry Consensus Conference Report, 2016. http://surgicalexcellence.org/wp-content/uploads/2017/04/ROBOTIC-REGISTRY-CONSENSUS-CONFERENCE-Summary-Report-10-23-16.pdf.

[13] Gaba DM. "The future vision of simulation in health care." *Quality and Safety in Health Care* 13, no. 1 (2004): i2–10.

[14] Issenberg SB, McGaghie WC, Hart IR, et al. "Simulation technology for healthcare professional skills training and assessment." *JAMA* 282, no. 9 (1999): 861–6.

[15] da Vinci® Skills Simulator (dVSS). Mimic Technologies Inc. Seattle, WA. https://mimicsimulation.com/da-vinci-skills-simulator/ (accessed July 7, 2019).

[16] RobotiX Mentor—3D Systems. Littleton, CO. https://simbionix.com/simulators/robotix-mentor/ (accessed July 7, 2019).

[17] McDonough PS, Tausch TJ, Peterson AC, Brand TC. "Initial validation of the ProMIS surgical simulator as an objective measure of robotic task performance." *Journal of Robotic Surgery* 5, no. 3 (2011), 195–9. doi:10.1007/s11701-011-0256-9.

[18] Wass V, Van der Vleuten C, Shatzer J, Jones R. "Assessment of clinical competence." *Lancet* 357 (2001): 945–9.

[19] Hung AJ, Zehnder P, Patil MB, Cai J, Ng CK, Aron M, Gill IS, Desai MM. "Face, content and construct validity of a novel robotic surgery simulator." *Journal of Urology* 186, no. 3 (2011): 1019–24.

[20] Kelly DC, Margules AC, Kundavaram CR, et al. "Face, content, and construct validation of the da Vinci Skills Simulator." *Urology* 79, no. 5 (2012): 1068–72.

[21] Hertz AM, George EI, Vaccaro CM, Brand TC. "'Head to head' comparison of three state of the art virtuality robotic surgery simulators." *Military Surgical Symposium 2018*. Presentation MSS24, Seattle, WA.

[22] Liss MA, Abdelshehid C, Quach S, et al. "Validation, correlation, and comparison of the da Vinci Trainer™ and the da Vinci surgical skills simulator™ using the Mimic™ software for urologic robotic surgical education." *Journal of Endourology* 26, no. 12 (2012): 1629–34.

[23] Tanaka A, Graddy C, Simpson K, et al. "Robotic surgery simulation validity and usability comparative analysis." *Surgical Endoscopy* 30, no. 9 (2016): 3720–9.

[24] Whittaker G, Aydin A, Raison KN, et al. "Validation of the RobotiX Mentor robotic surgery simulator." *Journal of Endourology* 30, no. 3 (2016): 338–46.

[25] Hutchins AR, Manson RJ, Lerebours R, Farjat AE, Cox ML, Mann BP, Zani S. "Objective assessment of the early stages of the learning curve for the senhance surgical robotic system." *Journal of Surgical Education* (2018). doi:10.1016/j.jsurg.2018.06.026.

[26] Chen R, Rodrigues Armijo P, Krause C; SAGES Robotic Task Force, Siu KC, Oleynikov D. "A comprehensive review of robotic surgery curriculum and training for residents, fellows, and

postgraduate surgical education." *Surgical Endoscopy* (2019 Apr 5). doi: 10.1007/s00464-019-06775-1.

[27] Satava RM, Stefanidis D, LevyJS, et al. "Proving the effectiveness of the fundamentals of robotic surgery (FRS) skills curriculum a single-blinded, multispecialty, multi-institutional randomized control trial." *Annals of Surgery* (2019).

[28] Smith R, Patel V, Satava R. "Fundamentals of robotic surgery: a course of basic robotic surgery skills based upon a 14-society consensus template of outcomes measures and curriculum development." *International Journal of Medical Robotics and Computer Assisted Surgery* 10, no. 3 (2014): 379–84.

[29] Welcome to FRS. (n.d.). http://frsurgery.org/ (accessed July 18, 2019).

[30] Robotics Training Network. (n.d.). https://robotictraining.org/ (accessed July 18, 2019).

[31] Jones DB, Stefanidis D, Korndorffer JR, Dimick JB, Jacob BP, Schultz L, Scott DJ. "SAGES University Masters program: a structured curriculum for deliberate, lifelong learning." *Surgical Endoscopy* 31 (2017): 3061–71.

[32] Fundamental Skills of Robot-Assisted Surgery (2018). https ://www.roswe llpar k.org/ education/atlas-program/testingtraining/fundamental-skill s-robot-assisted surgery-FSRS (accessed July 18, 2019).

[33] Stegemann AP, Ahmed K, Syed JR, et al. "Fundamental skills of robotic surgery: a multi-institutional randomized controlled trial for validation of a simulation-based curriculum." *Urology* 81, no. 4 (2013): 767–4. doi:10.1016/j.urology.2012.12.033.

[34] *Intuitive Surgical da Vinci Training* (2017). https://www.intuitives surgical.com/training/ (accessed July 18, 2019).

[35] da Vinci® Training Passport Technology Training Pathway: Surgeon.

[36] Intuitive Surgical Inc. Skills Simulator for the da Vinci SI Surgical System; 2012; da Vinci Skills Simulator; 2016. http://www.intuitivesurgical.com/products/ skills_simulator/ (accessed July 12, 2019).

[37] Marengo F, Larrain D, Babilonti L, et al. "Learning experience using the double-console da Vinci surgical system in gynecology: a prospective cohort study in a university hospital." *Archives of Gynecology and Obstetrics* 285 (2012): 441–5.

[38] Alemzadeh H, Raman J, Leveson N, Kalbarczyk Z, Iyer RK. "Adverse events in robotic surgery: a retrospective study of 14 years of FDA data." *PLoS One* 11, no. 4 (2016): e0151470. doi:10.1371/journal.pone.0151470.

[39] Robotic-Assisted Surgical Devices (RASD) CRN—MDEpiNet. *Medical Device Epidemiology Network*. http://mdepinet.org/rasd/ (accessed July 18, 2019).

[40] Fleurence RL, Shuren J. "Advances in the use of real-world evidence for medical devices: an update from the national evaluation system for health technology." *Clinical Pharmacology and Therapeutics* 106 (2019): 30–3. doi:10.1002/cpt.1380.

Grzegorz Cebula and Michał Nowakowski

12 Simulation in medical education—phantoms in medicine

12.1 Introduction

The dictionary prepared by the Society for Simulation in Healthcare has defined simulation as a technique that creates a situation or environment to allow persons to experience a representation of a real event for the purpose of practice, learning, evaluation, and testing or to gain understanding of systems or human actions [1].

Simulation plays an important role especially in the process of learning new skills. Thanks to the controlled environment, the learner has the opportunity to safely acquire and improve skills by repeating it without the consequences of potential error. Especially in medicine, this risk translates directly into the life and health of patients.

The optimal way to acquire complex skills is described by "the circle of learning." The process starts with the acquisition of knowledge related to a topic. Next in simulated conditions, the trainee acquires simple skills related to the implementation of the complete procedure. In the times of dynamic development of computer simulation, the next step might be an exercise based on computer programs or more advanced virtual reality techniques (serious gaming). The final stage of the simulation is to perform the task in conditions that reproduce as closely as possible an actual workplace (high-fidelity simulation).

A good example of such a process is learning how to perform cardiopulmonary resuscitation. Students first learn the knowledge necessary to understand the principles of resuscitation. Then, using simulators, they practice simple skills such as chest compressions, ventilation with a self-inflating bag and a face mask, securing airways procedure, intravascular access, ECG interpretation, and defibrillation. Procedures are learned separately, and the number of repetitions ensures mastery of basic skills. In the next stage, students might use computer programs simulating the work of the resuscitation team, in which students learn how to coordinate the work of members of the resuscitation team, control time, and carry out appropriate activities in accordance with the algorithm of advanced life support (ALS). Finally, the last stage is applying the principles of the reanimation team in simulated clinical settings where the additional difficulty is working in a real therapeutic team. Usually, at this stage, the group realizes that the ability to efficiently and correctly perform individual tasks detached from the whole task does not mean that the same procedures will be properly performed during more complex activities, i.e., in this case, the work of the resuscitation team performing a relatively uncomplicated ALS algorithm. Simulated clinical conditions allow the acquisition of new skills such as communication in a therapeutic team, team management, work as a team member, therapeutic decisions, and situation awareness.

12.2 Full-body simulators application in the training of medical personnel

12.2.1 History

The first full-body simulators were used in the education of nurses at the beginning of the 20th century. In 1911, the first full-length simulator was produced, which intends to be used to learn nurses' patient care [2]. Hartford Hospital approached the Rhode Island doll manufacturer M.J. Chase Co. to design the first manikin tailored for health care practice. Modeled and named after her creator, Martha Jenks Chase, Mrs. Chase since then, patient simulators have permanently found their place in laboratories where the basics skills of nursing were taught. The next step in the development of patient simulators was the publication of the articles that describe the standards of doing modern cardiopulmonary resuscitation and the creation of the first simulators designed to learn these skills in the 1950s by professors Peter Safar, William Kouwenhoven, and their collaborators. With the development of computers, simulators became more and more complex. They enable students to learn relatively simple skills such as patient care or chest compressions and ventilation. The first, computer-controlled, advanced patient simulator was developed in 1969 Sim One [3]. The mannequin replicated physiologic responses such as chest movement in respiration, blinking eyes, and pupils that have opened and closed. Sim One also had heartbeat, temporal and carotid pulse, and blood pressure. The simulator was developed by Dr. Stephen Abrahamson and Dr. Judson Denson and their team. The simulator was originally meant to be used mainly to train anesthesiologists. At the end of the 1980s, the next generation of patient simulators, controlled by PC computers, appeared. MedSim Eagle from 1986 already had almost all functions currently available in modern patient simulators: the ability to auscultate heart tones and respiratory murmurs, speaking with the help of a built-in loudspeaker and advanced hemodynamic monitoring. The further development of patient simulators was closely related to the development of computers, the miniaturization of equipment necessary to control, and the function of the simulator or wireless communication. Modern patient simulators are advanced robots that enable both history taking and physical examination of the simulated patient as well as performing numerous invasive procedures.

In this way, three basic types of full-body patient simulators were created to teach patient care, advanced cardiopulmonary resuscitation, and advanced patient simulators that you can use for clinical simulated scenarios.

12.3 The capabilities of different types of simulators

As mentioned before, technical skills training led to the development of full and partial body simulators. They remain the main way to improve technical competence in health care until today. There are some changes, mainly in the technical side of the hardware and software, but the main idea remains the same.

There is a vast number of simulators available commercially and more are in the development. As assessed in 2014 by Stunt et al. [4], there are more than 400 devices on the market excluding those used for demonstration purposes or knowledge transfer.

The basic principle is that we replace the whole body or a part of the body of the patient with an artificial device mimicking representative qualities. Because this chapter is devoted mostly to full-body simulators, we will concentrate on those. Partial body simulators will be mentioned only briefly to create a context.

12.3.1 Partial body simulators

They range from simulated skin pads to torso with or without head. Skin pads are used to teach/learn subcutaneous injections or skin incision, small excisions, and stitching. Slightly more elaborate simulators would depict part of the body like a limb or buttock to train intravenous (IV) access or intramuscular injections. All those simple task trainers can be either very simple or fairly complicated devices with lots of electronics or complicated mechanical or hydraulic parts to either give feedback on the quality of performance or to better emulate the reality. Hydraulics may include pipes representing venous or arterial vessels, urinary tract, or airways. They may depict normal body parts or pathological like fluid or air collections in chest drainage task trainers.

Feedback given by devices can also range from none to very elaborated assessment of quality of performance. Basic feedback can be delivered by simulated aspiration of air or artificial blood as a way to prove acceptable performance. More advance models may serve similar purposes but be as complicated and technologically advance as virtual reality injection simulator [5]. They provide numerical feedback on many aspects of performance, which may include but are not limited to timing, range of movement, or its linear or angular velocity. Of course, there are some models available, which provide some feedback related to set standards. Be it in the form of color-coded feedback (i.e., green for good, red for suboptimal performance) or any form of numerical or graphical representation.

One should also mention that some of the partial body simulators are meant as stand-alone devices while others as wearables enabling hybrid simulation with use of simulated/standardized patient (trained actor/lay person/patient) and partial body simulator at the same time. Examples would include wearable injection pads, breast models for physical examination, or even a full torso vest, enabling abdominal or thoracic surgical procedures in real time with blood pumping devices and artificial internal organs [6].

All the above-mentioned simulators are meant to give the caregiver a chance to perform tasks as closely resembling his/her future job as possible. However, there is also a need for empathy development, not only for technical skills enhancement. Here simulators help too. These are almost always wearables aimed at simulating different impairments so that future health care providers can experience limitations of handicapped people and thus understand them better and possibly identify a bit more with them building up the empathy and providing more emotion oriented care. These would include age simulators, eyesight, or hearing impairment simulators, pregnancy simulators, and many others.

Examples of partial body simulators include but are certainly not limited to the following:
- skin flaps to practice small surgical skills, suturing, and injections
- arm and forearm with hand for IV access
- head and neck for airways management
- upper torso and neck for large blood vessel access
- torso for pleural drainage or pneumothorax decompression
- legs for immobilization
- shins and arms or isolated respective bone structures for intraosseous access
- eyes and year to practice examination
- different body parts for decubitus management, bandaging and wound debridement, and dressing
- stoma care trainers (ileostomy, colostomy, urostomy, and gastrostomy)
- patient handicaps simulation (aging, eyesight and hearing loss, pregnancy, etc.)
- wearable simulators

12.3.2 Nursing care simulators

Nursing care simulators are designed mainly to teach technical skills that nurses should learn to properly care for patients, in particular, learning invasive procedures. Mastering such skills in the first place on simulators increases the safety of patients because the nurse for the first time performing a given procedure in a hospital setting has already acquired the basic skills at the simulation center.

Essential components of nursing care simulators are as follows:
- Full mobility of the joints and the body allowing simulate of real human movements
- Possibility to set the simulator in a lying and sitting position
- Anatomical points palpable for proper application of patient care (e.g., collarbone, sternum, and pelvic bones)
- Weight close to the weight of a real patient
- The ability to perform care procedures, such as
    - rinsing and cleaning the ears
    - removable dentures for learning oral hygiene and dentures
    - inserting the nasogastric tube and gastric lavage
    - tracheostomy care and suction from the respiratory tract
    - performing intravascular access, intramuscular, subcutaneous, and intradermal injections
    - intravenous medication and fluid infusion

- care of the vascular port, central venous access, etc.
- care for gastrostomy, colostomy, and nephrostomy
- bladder catheterization
- enema training
- measurement of blood pressure
- other

Most of these skills can be trained on task trainers, and in some learning situations, it is important to perform with a range of procedures on the same mannequin. Learning on full-body simulators increases the realism of simulation and allows participants to combine several different skills while training the care of a simulated patient, including nontechnical skills and teamwork.

12.3.3 Advances life support full-body simulator essential properties

The knowledge and skills of cardiopulmonary resuscitation is an important element of the medical staff training process. Every person working on patients should have at least basic resuscitation skills. Simulators from this group enable learning both basic and ALS skills.

The essential components of basic life support simulator are as follows:
- Lifelike anatomy allowing learning resuscitation
  - Perform nose-pinch, head tilt, chin lift, and jaw thrust
  - Ventilation (mouth to mouth, mouth to nose, self-inflating bag)
  - Chest compressions
- System designed to provide information about the quality of resuscitation might include several parameters, including but not limited to the following:
  - Ventilation volume
  - Correct ventilation percentage
  - Chest compressions depth
  - Chest compressions frequency
  - Correct chest compressions percentage
  - Compression to relaxation ratio
  - Information about wrong hands positioning on patient chest

In addition, advanced support simulator should include elements that enable additional procedures:
- Advanced airway management skills
- ECG monitoring and interpretation
- Defibrillation
- IV line insertion
- IV medicaments injections

That kind of equipment is used in training the resuscitation skills of teams and allows them to perform all standard procedures included in the ALS protocol.

12.3.4 Advanced patient simulators

Simulators of this type are used during high-fidelity simulations. High-fidelity simulation is defined as experiences that are extremely realistic and provide a high level of interactivity and realism for the learner.

These simulators usually include all functions that are incorporated to ALS training manikins. Components of advanced patient simulators might vary and depend mainly on simulator price. During exercises with an advanced patient simulator, the team usually is able to perform the following:
–   Securing airways using simple and advanced airway devices, including intubation and cricothyroidotomy
–   Suction oral cavity and airways
–   Oxygen therapy
–   Ventilation using bag valve mask or ventilator
–   IV or IO line insertion
–   Medicament infusion
–   Blood pressure measurement
–   Advanced vital signs monitoring (including SpO_2, $ETCO_2$, invasive BP, etc.)
–   Urethral catheterization
–   Chest needle decompression
–   Chest drain insertion

Patient simulator also allows physical examination and assessment of the following:
–   Risk of airway edema
–   Breathing rate
–   Chest wall movement
–   Lung sounds
–   Heart sounds
–   Bowel sounds
–   Pulse on central (carotid and femoral) and peripheral (radial) arteries
–   Pupils reaction to light
–   Skin moisture
–   Fluid leakage from ears, nose, mouth, and eyes

This type of simulator is most often used to learn teamwork in life-threatening situations of the patient, when it is necessary to perform numerous interventions, including invasive procedures, at the same time. High-fidelity simulation is also used to learn nontechnical skills.

12.3.5 Virtual reality and enhanced reality simulators

Technically speaking, they are not full-body simulators because per definition in virtual reality, there is no physical equipment at all (except from the computer and some sort of optical system), and for enhanced reality simulators, body parts are mostly simple plastic dolls. However, if we approach the topic cognitively by asking what sort of the work they do and what competencies they help to develop, it becomes clear that they belong to this section.

12.3.5.1 Virtual reality

These simulators take trainees to a nonexistent reality, which helps them to develop skills based on some simulation of respective sensory input. The most obvious one is visual simulation by means of monitors, goggles, or helmets. In the gaming industry, these also provide some sensory information by means of force feedback with especially designed vests. In medical training, force feedback is mostly limited to virtual reality surgical simulations, where force feedback simulates interaction between surgical tools and body parts or instrument collisions [7, 8].

There are numbers of uses for these devices. Developers reproduced almost all basic laparoscopic skill drills and a number of surgical procedures. The experience is still very different from reality, but research proves them to be effective training tools. The pricing of these devices is still a limiting factor, but that will probably be resolved in the future with market expansion and technological advances in consumer market. One unique feature of virtual reality surgical simulators is their ability to assist procedural training (not drills and basic skills only). The trainee can practice steps of real procedure in a gamelike fashion. These include but are not limited to laparoscopic cholecystectomy, gynecological laparoscopic procedures, or colorectal surgery. Apart from laparoscopy, a number of other virtual reality training tools are available on the market. Open orthopedic surgery VR trainers (some with tactile feedback delivered via VR gloves), arthroscopy, neurosurgery, maxilla-facial surgery, spine surgery, or endovascular surgery are the examples of disciplines where VR has a strong foothold. The number of these disciplines and available products grows daily. Advanced surgical manipulators (often called surgical robots) also have their respective simulators, making it certainly easier to transfer skills from open or laparoscopic surgery to robotic cases [9, 10].

12.3.5.2 Enhanced/augmented reality

Physical interaction with reality is very difficult to simulate virtually. It would require full-body suites with sensory input for tactile, pressure (weight), auditory, and visual stimuli. By contrast, physical simulators lack reality in some aspects like human-human interaction, nonverbal communication, face mimics, or movement. It is also very time consuming to moulage (apply characterization makeup) the physical simulators. It is also a very big organizational effort to simulate the environment that plays a key role in high-fidelity, ultrarealistic training.

Here enhanced reality originally introduced for military purposes (Virtual Fixtures for U.S. Air Force) later made its way to other industries, including fashion, sales, e-commerce, advertisement, transportation (augmented reality navigation systems), education, and health care. The obvious reasons are that it could possibly take the best of both worlds. Tactile, proprioceptive (positional), and partially audio and visual sensory input could be supplemented with additional sensory information. Currently, it is mostly visual because of the dominance of that sensory mode in humans, but other senses that are experimented with include smell or audio [11–13].

The modes of delivery of these modified sensory inputs are numerous, and they include head-mounted eye glasses, helmets, goggles, direct retina display devices, and others. One must also remember that sometimes it is the group rather than the single user that needs to have sensory input modified. For this situation, spatial augmented reality systems are developed, and they include projectors, lights, speakers, and smoke simulators to modify the environment rather than the single user sensory input.

12.4 Nontechnical skills training

The aim of this chapter was to shortly present topics related to training in the field of nontechnical skills for people working in therapeutic teams (trauma team, resuscitation team, etc.). This type of exercise should be a compulsory part of the curriculum of medical students and postgraduate training, not only doctors but also nurses, midwives, paramedics, and other people who in the future after graduation will operate in the conditions of a multispecialized therapeutic team.

12.4.1 Crisis resource management

Crisis resource management (CRM) is a set of procedures and rules for use in environments where human error may have disastrous consequences. It enables the optimal use of all available resources (people, procedures, and equipment), which increase the safety and effectiveness of actions in a crisis, thanks to the decreasing numbers of errors due to the human factor [1].

Human factor is the discipline or science of studying the interaction between humans and systems and technology; it includes, but is not limited to, principles and applications in the areas of human engineering, personnel selection, training, life support, job performance aids, and human performance evaluation (M&S Glossary) [1].

Creating the basic principles of CRM, you can base yourself on the following skill list:
- Situation awareness
- Planning and decision making

- Teamwork skills
- Team leader skills
- Communication

12.4.1.1 Situation awareness

Situation awareness is the ability to continuously collect data from the environment in relation to the situation in which a person is located, enabling the identification and interpretation of changes taking place in the environment and predicting their effect in the near future.

In short, this means seeing and knowing what's going on and predicting what's going to happen next.

The three elements/levels of situational awareness are as follows [14]:
- Perception of elements of the current situation
- Understanding/creating an image of the current situation (mental model)
- Anticipating options that will be possible in the near future/what will happen in a moment

12.4.1.2 Cognitive errors

Problems at any of the three stages of creating situation awareness can cause a cognitive error. As a result of incorrect data collection or interpretation, the team make decisions and takes actions that are inadequate to the situation.

When investigating adverse events in aviation, Mc Carthy stated that the occurrence of a cognitive error usually occurs in situations when [15]
- the attention is too focused, which in effect leads to receiving only a part of the information—31% of the investigated events;
- the attention is dispersed by factors unrelated to the task being performed—22% of the investigated events;
- the tasks performed are too complicated to the level of training of people participating in it—17% of investigated events;
- the team focuses on one activity and omits or refrains from performing other tasks important from the point of view of patient safety—17% of the investigated events.

This leads to dangerous situations. The doctor may be convinced that he has made a correct diagnosis and started treating the patient, although the cause of the problem is completely different (this and only this).

In the case of a fixation error such as "all but not this," the doctor takes into account several possible options but excluding one as impossible, usually out of fear of its consequences.

Another relatively common cognitive error includes the situation on the team's conviction about the absence of a threat, although the situation requires immediate action to overcome the actual real life or health threat (everything is fine). A typical example of this situation is an adverse event described in the YouTube movie *Just*

Routine Operation, where the lack of situation awareness was one of elements of an adverse event that led to the patient's death as a result of hypoxia.

12.4.1.3 Planning and decision making

Decision making is a process of gathering and processing information, which results in a nonrandom selection of one solution to the problem from at least two or more available solutions. The decision-making process has been in the field of interest for both scientists and practitioners for many years. The effect of this was the development of tools to facilitate the decision-making process.

Typically, decision making involves successive actions as follows:

- Assessment of the situation
- Development and consideration of one or more action options, selection of one option
- Implementation of the decision
- Evaluation of the effects of the action taken and implemented

One of the ways to support the decision-making process is to describe the next steps of the process with the letters of the acronym, e.g., the DODAR acronym used by British Airways pilots:

D, detect—We detect the problem. The patient's blood pressure falls.
I should collect data. When was the last time this parameter was observed/measured? What happens to other vital signs? (Does the respiration rate increase or decrease?) The monitor may have broken down or the measuring cuff has moved—it must be "detected."
What are the possible reasons for this situation? What have we done to prevent it so far?

O, options—In understanding the problem, we have to consider options.
We consider possible options together with the team. What are the possibilities of conduct? How do you find the cause of the pressure drop? How do you treat a patient?

D, decision—We make a decision.
As the person managing the team, we must decide at some point what we are going to do, what is the plan.

A, actions/assignments—These are tasks/work assignments.
We inform the team what the plan is about and what we will do. We will share tasks.

R, review—When the plan is implemented, at the first opportunity, when we have a few seconds break, we are reviewing the situation. Did we remember everything? What else can you do?

12.4.2 Teamwork

Management of patient in a life-threatening situation usually requires the work of a team of people. The team consists of people with different experiences, skills, and abilities working together to increase the chance of effective treatment of the patient.

Proper teamwork can have a significant effect on the final result of patient treatment.

What makes a team efficient?
–   Individual team member's skills
–   Proper task distribution
–   Work coordination
–   Good team leader
–   Communication skills
–   Motivation

12.4.2.1 The 10-seconds-for-10-minutes technique—sharing decision making

Working in a team gives a unique opportunity to use the knowledge and skills of all group members during the decision-making process. This action has certain consequences. Lack of information may result in different, often contradictory, ways of solving the problem they are experiencing by different team members.

Passing all the necessary information to all team members might require a short break in activities (stop) [16], during which team members share their information and jointly conduct an assessment of the situation. The effect of such an exchange of views should be to jointly establish a list of problems that the team encounters at a given moment, set priorities, and decide on actions to be taken in the near future.

It is true that ultimately the team leader will accept the decisions made, but at the same time, it should be remembered that obedience to the superior, an excessive desire to please others, and giving someone else's opinion over their own could lead to an adverse event.

12.4.2.2 Team leader skills

Team leaders appear everywhere where groups of people are used to carry out tasks. One of their main tasks is to ensure the effective functioning of the team.

A team leader is a formally or informally chosen person whose tasks consist of
–   management and coordination,
–   motivating to work together,
–   evaluation of activities,
–   planning and organization of work—setting priorities,
–   ensuring a good atmosphere in the team [17].

12.4.2.3 Communication

Communication in large part is responsible for the correct teamwork, somehow linking all the previously described elements. It is defined as transmitting and receiving information between two or more people. We can also define communication by answering four questions:
- What—information transfer
- How—the way communication is conducted
- Why—the reason for communication
- Who—communicating persons

During simulation, we can teach participants how to communicate properly and give them few relatively easy skills that make communication better.

12.4.2.4 Close loop communication

Close loop communication involves interaction between the sender and the recipient. In this system, the person who is the recipient of the information processes it and then transfers it back to the sender.

Example:
Team leader: Piotr, inject 1 mg of adrenaline intravenously.
Piotr (team member): I'm going to give 1 mg of adrenaline intravenously.

Such a way of communicating may take a bit more time, but it is more effective and safe. The sender is calmer hearing the feedback from the recipient. The recipient also feels more confident knowing that the sender has checked whether he has properly heard and understood the information.

12.4.2.5 Team member's name use during communication

The message may not reach the team member simply because he is not expecting it, he is busy carrying out ordered tasks, or he is wondering how to optimally solve the situation. The reason for the failure to perform the task may also be in the way it is formulated; for example, the "we should give morphine" command will most probably not be done because it is not known to whom it is addressed or can be interpreted as a question of opinion or thinking aloud. When formulating requests or commands, you should always start them with the name of the person to whom the message is addressed, and it may be accompanied by nonverbal communication (e.g., looking at him, touching him); e.g., Piotr, give 1 mg of adrenaline intravenously.

12.4.2.6 Team assertiveness

Each team member should be able to speak their opinion openly, also when their point of view does not agree with the team leader's point of view. The ability to take such a tactful and effective message is crucial to the safety of teamwork.

The message "I think we are going a bit too low" may not have the proper effect when the plane is several dozen meters above the ground and height continues to decrease.

In simple situations in which the decision of the team leader is in conflict with the organization of work in the ward or guidelines, the question "Are you sure?" might be enough to correct a decision. If there is no reaction, you can take further steps to solve the problem. Constructing subsequent statements can be based on proven assertiveness grading schemes such as CUSS or PACE.

CUSS
- C, concern—I am concerned that ...
- U, unsure—I'm not sure that ...
- S, safety—It is not safe.
- S, stop—Stop it immediately.

PACE
- P, probe—Did you know ...? I do not understand why you want to do it.
- A, alert (vigilance)—I think that your decisions will cause ...
- C, challenge—Your actions will hurt because ...
- E, emergency action—Stop it immediately! For the sake of the patient, we should ...

12.4.3 Technical skills training

As mentioned previously, technical skills training led to the development of full and partial body simulators. They remain the main way to improve technical competence in health care until today, and they are very likely to stay with us much longer. There are some changes, mainly in the technical side of the hardware and software, but the main idea remains the same.

The basic principle is that we replace the whole body or a part of the body of the patient with an artificial device mimicking representative qualities. Because this chapter is devoted mostly to full-body simulators, we will concentrate on those.

The basic principle of training of any technical skill with any sort of simulator is that the costs of training (understood not as monetary costs but also as organizational costs, risk management, possibility of injury to the trainee or the subject of procedure, cognitive and emotional challenges, and all possible other material or immaterial costs) must be lowered so that it makes training easier to be applied many times to increase the performance in real situation. One must also keep in mind that the frequency of utilization of a particular skill in real life must be taken into consideration. For these rarely performed tasks requiring high skills, simulation might be the only method to achieve competence. An easy example comes from the aviation industry: emergency landing procedures in case of failure of some of aircraft's systems is better not to be practiced first time in reality with 335 passengers on board Boeing 787 Dreamliner. It is possible to reliably simulate these events on demand in a safe training environment. The same principle is applied in medicine. Some of the most widespread examples are BLS and ALS training programs. Majority of trained personnel will not perform practiced skills at all or will do that very rarely, making simulation the main way to acquire and maintain the skills.

Safety consideration applies to both sides of that equitation. Simulation-based training makes personnel more technically apt but also gives the trainees so much needed self-confidence and possibility to avoid putting ones training above the safety of patients [18].

As far as utilization of training devices go, a typical approach is to use step-up training modes. Initially, trainees receive information (knowledge transfer) on how a procedure should be performed. That is passed by means of live or recorded demonstration, text, drawings, or any other way known in knowledge transfer. The second step includes explanation of optimal performance, and the third step includes one practice preferably with some sort of feedback or correction from the trainer. Several methodologies have been developed to enhance the effectiveness of training [19].

12.4.3.1 See one, do one, teach one

It is one of the most popular and also one of worst understood modalities. Often incorrectly used as a synonym of an easy task as in "this is so easy you can have a look once, then you can do it alone and next time you can teach it." The real reasoning behind this method is that you need to see something done first, and then you should do it yourself; once you are able to teach it, that is when you really know how to do it. For simple tasks, it is really effective and it also improves trainee engagement because they are given bigger responsibilities. The ability to teach in this case means not pedagogical skills but sufficient understanding and proper acquisition of manual competence to demonstrate and explain.

12.4.3.2 Peyton four-step approach

Based on cognitive sciences, a system for the optimization of technical skills transfer has been developed [20]. It is a bit more elaborate and probably more effective. It includes four steps:
1. Demonstration
2. Deconstruction
3. Comprehension
4. Execution

In the first step, students should observe a real-time, real-speed demonstration of good quality performance without any distraction, breaks, or explanations. The reason is for students to be able to have a clear reference regarding the expected standard of performance.

In the second step, students should see the procedure one more time, but this time with comments and explanations. This step is meant to clarify all doubts, explain the crucial moments, and point out crucial steps.

In the third step, students should aim at understanding all steps and ways to perform. In reality, it is often done in a way that while an instructor performs a third demonstration, one of students describes the crucial steps.

In the fourth step, the student performs by himself. This step can be used for the next student to perform step 3.

This sequence enables the utilization of different modalities of learning. In the first step, it is visualization and time stamping (realization of timing of the procedure). In the second step, it is auditory learning. The third step is verbalization, and the fourth one is using kinesthetic memorization.

Peyton's four-step approach requires careful planning of the teaching session. First, a skill to be taught must not take too long to demonstrate. Simple technical procedures like BLS, IV line placement, or simple airway management are most commonly taught that way. Second, it is important to think through your explanations carefully. What is done in step 2 must not be too complicated, should be easy to remember, and should easily trigger the next step. It is meant to help students perform, and he/she must remember it at one go. If the procedure needs more explanations, either it is not the best choice for this method or the explanation should take place in a form of lecture or other knowledge transfer method before skill practice.

The model is flexible enough that it can be adapted to other tasks. It is being used (intentionally or not) in training some complex technical skills like surgery. For the first few cases, the trainee observes, receives explanation, asks and answers questions, does probe understanding, and then finally performs. This is just but one modification of numerous published practices throughout the world.

12.4.3.3 Slicing method/skill deconstruction

Some fairly complicated tasks are difficult to teach, especially to larger (5–20) groups of trainees when demonstrated and explained. One needs to break them into much smaller, "digestible" parts. It is usually one specific move that is being demonstrated after another. It helps to have them named ("word coded"). Individual moves are merged into sequences and then whole tasks. A useful analogy would be teaching dancing. First, trainees learn steps, then figures, then predefined choreography, and only then they improvise.

That method can be easily adapted to teaching larger groups of people with diverse starting points or different manual dexterity. Slices are cut down to the level of the person with the lowest skill and tempo of progress to the level of the slowest learner. That way, the whole group can be taught with limited resources, but of course the potential of the fastest learners or people with the highest skill on entry is not used properly.

12.4.3.4 Programmatic teaching of technical skills

It is important to plan skill acquisition into the course, the subject, or the whole training curriculum. It is known that teaching in any domain (knowledge, technical, or nontechnical skills) is best done when new competencies are built on the previous ones. This helps retention and increases the tempo of acquisition. It is of course no different for technical skills. Most teachers agree on the step-up approach. The trainee starts with small, isolated skills and then merges into more complex tasks to progress to full procedures. Often, this step is followed by merging several procedures to be performed in proper sequence. At different stages, some nontechnical skills are usually blended because technical competence alone is very often not sufficient in today's world. Training of these nontechnical competences has been described in Chapter 12.4.

The typical sequence could include a simple station to teach an assembly of IV access kit followed by a task trainer (an IV access arm). Once students are reasonably fluent with this, an advanced full-body simulator and a simple clinical scenario where students have to perform an IV access can be used. Later stages may include a hybrid simulation with IV access after they explain the procedure and obtain informed consent form a simulated patient to finally arrive to a high-fidelity simulation where IV access is but a small task within reach simulated workplace experience.

This progress in training is essential to keep students' engagement at high levels and also to properly adjust the level of training to trainees' abilities and needs.

12.5 Summary

Full and partial body simulators as well as virtual and augmented reality simulation in medical education are a cornerstone of modern training programs. They help to increase patients' and trainees' safety and also lower the costs of training and increase its effectiveness. Current trends produce more advanced equipment in all ranges of simulators, from the basic ones to the most complex, hybrid teaching environments. Teaching both technical and nontechnical skills is essential, and it can often be done in a close sequence using similar methodologies and equipment. In the future, we will probably see much more of that technological progress, especially in the field of virtual and augmented reality simulators.

12.6 References

[1] Lopreiato JO, Downing D, Gammon W, Lioce L, et al. *Healthcare Simulation Dictionary*. https://www.ssih.org/Dictionary

[2] Grypma S. "In retrospect: regarding Mrs. Chase." *Journal of Christian Nursing* 29, no. 3 (July/September 2012): 181.

[3] Abrahamson S, Wolf RM, Denson JS. "A computer-based patient simulator for training anaesthesiologists." *Educational Technology* 9 (October 1969): 55–9.

[4] Stunt J, Wulms P, Kerkhoffs G, Dankelman J, van Dijk C, Tuijthof G. "How valid are commercially available medical simulators?" *Advances in Medical Education and Practice* 5 (2014): 385–95.

[5] McWilliams LA, Malecha A. "Comparing intravenous insertion instructional methods with haptic simulators." *Nursing Research and Practice* 2017 (2017): 4685157.

[6] Kirkpatrick AW, Tien H, LaPorta AT, et al. "The marriage of surgical simulation and telementoring for damage-control surgical training of operational first responders: a pilot study." *Journal of Trauma and Acute Care Surgery* 79 no. 5 (2015): 741–7.

[7] Botden SM, Buzink SN, Schijven MP, Jakimowicz JJ. "Augmented versus virtual reality laparoscopic simulation: what is the difference? A comparison of the ProMIS augmented reality laparoscopic simulator versus LapSim virtual reality laparoscopic simulator." *World Journal of Surgery* 31, no. 4 (2007): 764–72.

[8] Zhou M, Tse S, Derevianko A, Jones DB, Schwaitzberg SD, Cao CG. "Effect of haptic feedback in laparoscopic surgery skill acquisition." *Surgical Endoscopy* 26, no. 4 (2012): 1128–34.

[9] Sun AJ, Aron M, Hung AJ. "Novel training methods for robotic surgery." *Indian Journal of Urology* 30, no. 3 (2014): 333–8.

[10] Foell K, Finelli A, Yasufuku K, et al. "Robotic surgery basic skills training: evaluation of a pilot multidisciplinary simulation-based curriculum." *Canadian Urological Association Journal* 7, nos. 11–12 (2013): 430–4.

[11] Munzer BW, Khan MM, Shipman B, Mahajan P. "Augmented reality in emergency medicine: a scoping review." *Journal of Medical Internet Research* 21 no. 4 (2019): e12368. Published 2019 Apr 17.

[12] Vávra P, Roman J, Zonča P, et al. "Recent development of augmented reality in surgery: a review." *Journal of Healthcare Engineering* 2017 (2017): 4574172. doi:10.1155/2017/4574172.

[13] Riva G, Wiederhold BK, Mantovani F. "Neuroscience of virtual reality: from virtual exposure to embodied medicine." *Cyberpsychology, Behavior, and Social Networking* 22, no. 1 (2019): 82–96.

[14] Endsley MR. "Toward a theory of situation awareness in dynamic systems." *Human Factors* 37, no. 1 (1995): 32–64.

[15] Mc Carthy, GW. "Human factors in F-16 mishaps." *Flying Safety* (May 1988).

[16] Rall M, Glavin RJ. "The '10-seconds-for-10-minutes' principle. Why things go wrong and stopping them getting worse." *Bulletin of the Royal College of Anaesthetists* 51 (September 2008).

[17] Day DV, Zaccaro SJ, Halpin SM. *Leader Development for Transforming Organizations: Growing Leaders for Tomorrow.* 1st ed. Psychology Press, January 2004.

[18] Maxwell WD, Mohorn PL, Haney JS, et al. "Impact of an advanced cardiac life support simulation laboratory experience on pharmacy student confidence and knowledge." *American Journal of Pharmaceutical Education* 80, no. 8 (2016): 140. doi:10.5688/ajpe8081400.

[19] van de Mortel TF, Silberberg PL, Ahern CM, Pit SW. "Supporting near-peer teaching in general practice: a national survey." *BMC Medical Education* 16 (2016): 143. Published 2016 May 12.

[20] Krautter M, Dittrich R, Safi A, et al. "Peyton's four-step approach: differential effects of single instructional steps on procedural and memory performance—a clarification study." *Advances in Medical Education and Practice* 6 (2015): 399–406. Published 2015 May 27.

Index

3D 109
3D4Medical 56
3D bioprinting 11
3D dose distributions 136
3D models 110
3D printing 4, 5, 63, 64, 65, 67, 69, 70, 71
3D virtual operating 86

anchors 92
animation 55
application 114
articulated arm 133
artificial 105
artificial intelligence 92
artificial reality 73
astigmatism 61
Atrial fibrillation 100
augmented reality (AR) 9, 10, 11, 73, 104, 154, 183
augmented visualization 111
automatic control 137
auxiliary elements 135

bedside assistance 159
biclustering 3
bioprinting 4
box trainers 157
brachytherapy 148
Brainstorm 47

calibration tools 133
cardiac interventions 96
cardiopulmonary bypass 95
C-arm 96
choreography 81
circle of learning 168
collection of waste 136
colorimetric tests 6
computer simulation 168
Conflict 77
console 86
console training 159
coronary artery bypass grafting 99
correlates of emotion 19, 27
Cox-Maze procedure 100

Crisis resource management 175
cyberknife 135
cyberspace 73
cytotoxic drugs 136

database of contractors 143
Data Matrix 139
da Vinci 119, 120, 123, 124, 125
da Vinci surgical robotic system 152
DEAP 23, 24, 25, 28
Deciding 77
decision-making 63, 67, 77, 175, 177
decision-making process 77, 78
dedicated containers 136
degrees of freedom 76
demographics data 140
Determined 77
device data 162
device malfunction 162
diagnostic 74
DICOM RT 137
Digital 105
Dipole source modeling 39
dominant rhythms 38
dorsal elevation 83
drag and drop 57
drug design 11
dual-console 161
dynamics 74

EEG lab 47
efficiency 78, 91
e-learning 55, 154
electric charge flowing 41
Electroencephalography 35
emotion correlates 20, 21
empathy 170, 171
endoscopic 88
endoscopic camera 131
endoscopic imaging 128
Endovascular aortic repair 100
enhanced reality 175
environment 106
ergonomics 76, 78
ERP 39

https://doi.org/10.1515/9783110667219-013

Event-related potentials 39
exercises 86
extended reality 9
extension arm 83
eyeball 57

FDA 70, 71, 153
FDA-approved surgical robotic devices 151
feedback 170
FLEX 123, 125
Foundation of Cardiac Surgery Development
    (Fundacja Rozwoju Kardiochirugrii im. Prof.
    Zbigniewa Religi [FRK]) 75
freezing the position of instruments 132
full-body simulators 172
Fundamentals of Laparoscopic Surgery
    (FLS) 150
Fundamentals of Robotic Surgery (FRS) 152
futuristic 105

General Data Protection Regulations 114
GeoSource 46
glasses 109

half-translucency 56
Heart Team 98
high-fidelity simulation 168, 173
high-quality video system 133
HoloAnatomy 109
hologram 6, 92, 103, 107, 111
holographic 103, 104, 106, 108, 109, 110, 112,
    113, 115
holography 104, 110, 112, 114
HoloLens 104, 106, 108, 109, 110, 112, 113,
    114, 115
home medicines 140
human eye 56
Human factor 175
hybrid 129
Hybrid coronary artery revascularization 99
hybrid models 91
hybrid operating room (OR) 9
hybrid OR 9, 11
hybrid procedures 95, 97
hybrid room 95, 97, 98, 128
hybrid specialists 98

ICA 42
image fusion 97

imaging 4, 5, 8, 9, 11, 110
imaging systems 128
immersive 107
importing/exporting data 148
Independent component analysis 42
individual processes 130
instrument arms 132
integration systems 129
intervention 90
intraoperative microscopes 128
invasiveness 90
invasive techniques 128
Iowa Gambling Task 48
IT 78

keyboard 132
kinematics 74

laparoscope 79
laparoscopic 76, 132
laparoscopic skill drills 174
laparoscopy 150
learning curve 77
liver surgery 66, 67
LORETA 40

manipulative 83
manual training 79
mechanical holder 133
mechanical probe 133
mechatronic 82, 86, 88
medical images 108
Mentoring 161
mesh 65
mini-invasive surgical methods 79
minimal invasive surgeries 7
minimally invasive surgery 150
Mixed Reality 108
modeling 5, 8, 10, 11, 74, 77
modules 134
multidrug pills 5
muscles 57
myopia 61

nerves 57
Net Station 44
neural network 22, 27, 28
neurofeedback 29
nontechnical skills 173, 183

nurses 169, 171, 175
nursing 169, 171
nursing staff 141

observation of robotic surgeries 154
OpenSesame 43
operating table, like in teleoperations, introduces responsibility problems because of 78
Operation 74
optical distance 133

P300 39
palm flexion 83
pathological anatomy 57
patient simulators 169
Peyton four-step approach 181
Peyton's four-step approach 182
physical modeling 79
physical simulators 157
Picture Archiving and Communication Systems 97
planning 74
platform 86
positioning 56
power spectrum 38
precision medicine 2, 6
principal component analysis 42
prognostic 74
proportions 56
psychomotor skills 158

Random 77
rare disease 3
Recognition 77
regulatory decision making 164
remote control operation 78
reoperation 73
repeatability 82
resting state 37
Robin Heart 75, 80, 81, 82, 85, 86
robot 75, 76, 81, 82, 85, 88, 90
robot-assisted surgery 7, 151
robotic 78, 82, 88
robotic instrument 131
Robotic optics 135
Robotic surgery 151
robotic surgery registry 162
robotization 138

safety and efficacy 153
segmentation 64, 69, 70
Senhance surgical robotic system 152
serious games 55
Simulated clinical conditions 168
simulated workplace 183
simulation 75, 76
simulation environments 155
single-choice questions 56
single player mode 55
Situation awareness 175, 176
sLORETA 40
smartphone 92
socket bone 57
Source localization 40
standardization 74, 82
strategy 74
stream of information 144
students' engagement 183
surface rendering 64
surgical robots 131
surgical simulations 174
Surgical workshop 89

task trainers 170, 172
TAVI 98
team leader 178
teamwork 173
technical 183
technical skill 169, 180
technical skills training 180
technologies 107
technology-saturated zone 129
telemanipulation 83
telemanipulator 75, 78, 83, 86, 88
telemedical system 86
teleoperation 77
training 77, 79, 80
training and credentialing 153
trocar point 135
two-dimensional bar code 139

unfolding into parts 56

virtual 183
virtual model 55, 88
virtual operating room 78
virtual reality (VR) 9, 10, 27, 73, 75, 79, 81, 82, 86, 90, 92, 104, 168

virtual space 75, 81, 90
visualization 8, 111
visualize anatomical structures 115
visual simulation 174
VR simulator platforms 155
VR technologies 76

wearable 170
workstation 86

XR 10